James Duigan's Blueprint for Health

James Duigan's Blueprint for Health

THE BODYISM
4 PILLARS
OF HEALTH

- MINDSET
- NUTRITION
- MOVEMENT
- SLEEP

First published in the United Kingdom in 2017 by
Pavilion
43 Great Ormond Street
London
WC1N 3HZ

ISBN 978-1-911216-64-3

A CIP catalogue record for this book is
available from the British Library.

10 9 8 7 6 5 4 3 2 1

Reproduction by Mission Productions, Hong Kong
Printed and bound by G. CANALE & C. S.p.A. Italy

This book can be ordered direct from
the publisher at www.pavilionbooks.com

CONTENTS

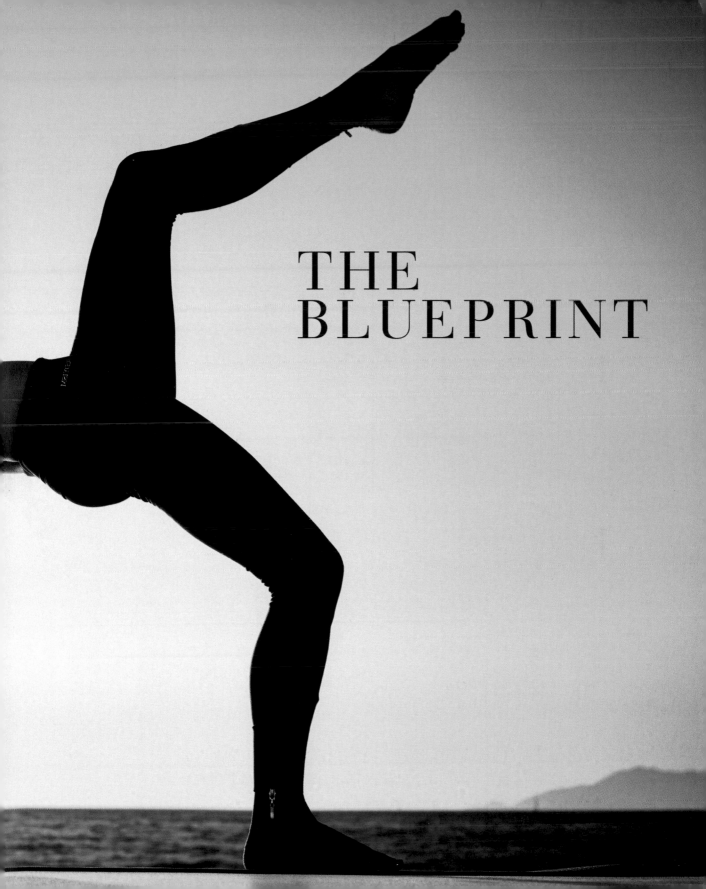

THE
BLUEPRINT

INTRODUCTION

'Be open to everything, to all possibilities, listen and be curious.' DR WAYNE DYER

Throughout history, four key pillars of health have been respected: mindset, nutrition, movement and sleep. But sadly, right now, living by these four pillars has never been more difficult to maintain. There are more ways to communicate than ever before, but we've never been lonelier. More food is being mass produced, but we've never been more malnourished. There is more research about the importance of sleep than ever before, but we've never been more sleep deprived. And gyms are popping up on every street corner, but we've never been less active. The Bodyism ethos is guided by the simple philosophy, 'Be kind to yourself'. No superfood, health trend or exercise class can do that for you, but by making positive changes to each of the four pillars of health, you can.

This is a really momentous point in my life because, as I write this book, I feel that I have finally found balance across all four pillars of health. If you don't feel balanced, I understand you, because I've been there. Over the years, even while writing bestselling books, running the most luxurious gym in the world and being at the forefront of the wellness industry, I have still struggled to get to grips with each of the four pillars. So don't beat yourself up, just return to our simple philosophy. This book will show you how to navigate today's world so you feel and look healthy, achieve your optimum state of wellness and learn to be truly kind to yourself.

Throughout this book (and for the rest of your life), look at the four pillars of health equally. See them like the tyres on your car. As you travel through your life, if one of those tyres is faulty or not quite aligned, eventually, over time, it will cause some issues.

The more out of alignment that tyre is, the bigger and more serious these issues become and the more quickly they will have an impact on each other. Just as we would pay equal attention to each tyre, we need to pay the same amount of attention to each pillar of health. When we make positive changes to each pillar, our overall sense of wellness will transform. It's time to change your life.

First, ask the right questions.

Why is it that diets don't work? Why is it that so many people fail in their pursuit of health? In large part, it is because people are looking for answers when they really need the right questions. Always start with your 'why'. 'Why do I want to lose weight?' 'Why do I want to eat well?' 'Why do I want to feel healthy?' My 'why' is 'Why do I want to live a long, healthy and happy life?' And my answer is 'To be a strong father for my kids (and one day grandkids)'. That 'why' keeps me focused on making the right decisions in all four pillars of health.

If you have picked this book up, you are already halfway there. You already want to make a change. You probably know why you want to make that change and now you are just trying to work out how you are going to do it. My Blueprint for Health will offer questions and answers to help you understand the importance of the four pillars and your connection to them. A word of warning: my intention is always to help. I want to be truthful. I don't want the message to get lost in diplomatic fluff. Choose not to be offended. Being offended is a waste of time. Take inspiration from Dr Wayne Dyer and choose to be curious.

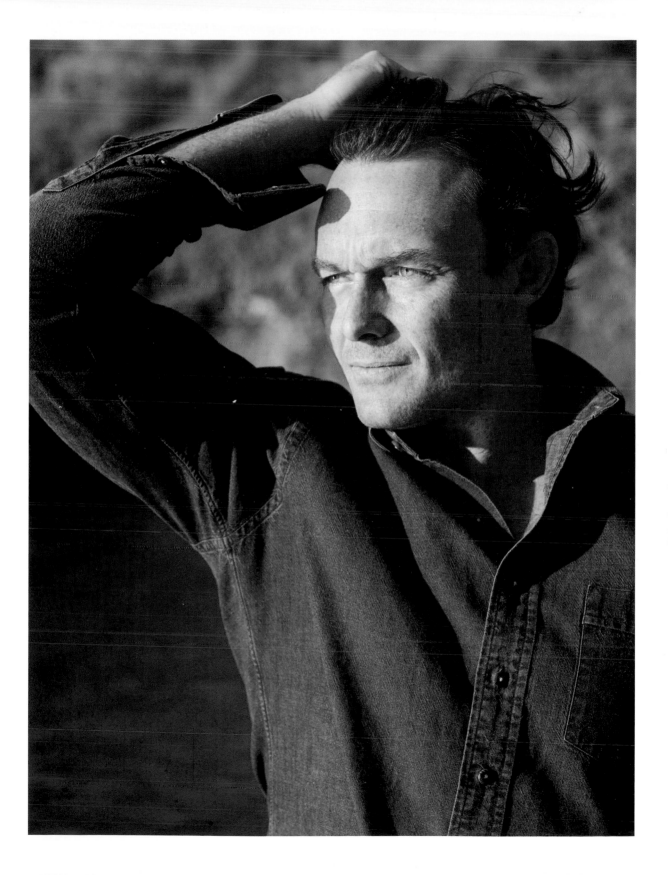

HOW DID I IDENTIFY THE 4 PILLARS?

Beware of the cat

My understanding of the four pillars began very early on in life. When I was five years old, I was hyperactive and had behavioural problems. I literally couldn't sit still, I was constantly in trouble at school, I couldn't sleep through the night and I remember the feeling of just not being comfortable in my own skin. My parents took me to a doctor who prescribed sedatives throughout the day to 'control' my behaviour, tranquilizers at night to 'help' me sleep and steroids to 'fix' my cough.

Even back then (35 years ago), my parents felt that was quite a heavy prescription of drugs; it seemed like a hell of a lot to put a tiny kid through.

Somehow, they managed to find a naturopath, Helen Neitzsche (I'll always remember her name). Her words were, 'Why don't we take him off sugar for a couple of weeks and see how that goes?' And, by the way, I wasn't eating anything out of the ordinary; I followed what was considered a 'normal' diet: a sugary breakfast cereal in the morning, with a glass of orange juice (because that was healthy); at morning break, a chocolate doughnut; at lunch, maybe a sandwich; I'd get home and have some chocolate milk; dinner would usually be a pre-made oven meal (this was the time when microwaves were only for super-fancy people) and then, for dessert, I'd have a bowl of ice cream with chocolate sauce. Looking back, this was a horrendous amount of sugar, but there simply wasn't the awareness back then that there is now. Bear in mind, the very fact that

you are reading this book means that you have at least some interest in health and wellness, but there are many people that would look at that diet and think it was absolutely fine — and wonder why they or their family are suffering from poor health.

My parents followed the naturopath's advice and made me cut out sugar, and, after three days, I was behaving like a normal person. I remember suddenly feeling calm rather than 'tired and wired', as I had felt constantly when I was completely high on sugar. And, by the way, at the end of that first week, our pet cat ran away and my cough disappeared. Yes, you guessed it: I was allergic to cats. If it wasn't for the doubt of my parents or the love of God (or whatever you choose to believe in), I could have been on the road to a drugged-up life of chemical addiction, sugar addiction and illness. So, very early on, I understood the very powerful connection between what you eat and how you feel. **That's how I identified the pillar of Nutrition.**

My fat story

When I was eight years old, I went to live in a place called Flying Fish Point, in Queensland. I barely went to school; I spent my days chasing butterflies, fishing, climbing trees and making stuff with whatever I could find in the rainforest. I picked fresh papayas, mangoes and avocados off the trees (a powerful health tip: eating anything freshly picked is one of the best things you'll ever do for your health and is one of the most powerful sources of probiotics you can get). I was so active, healthy and happy. Then I moved with my mum to Barnsley, in the north of England (to reconnect with my mum's northern-English roots) and had a culture shock. I spent my days watching 'Dallas' and 'Dynasty' and I slipped back into a toxic, high-sugar diet (more on what this means later). I felt awful and, for lack of a more diplomatic phrase, I got fat.

The first time I got any inkling that I had 'changed' was when I returned to Australia. My dad hadn't seen me for months (this was before the days of Facebook, Facetime and Skype). I remember him opening the door and he said, 'Bloody hell! What happened to you? You got fat.' He said it straight: 'Come on, mate, you need to sort it out.' I should say that my dad was the most gentle and loving person in the world. I'm sure what he said sounds harsh and, coming from anyone else it would have been, but he was such a gentle soul and he only knew how to speak the truth. I remember I didn't wait one minute. I put my bags down, tied the laces on my desert boots and went on a run around the block. That was the first time I realized how amazing the simple act of moving made me feel. I didn't wait for tomorrow to go on that run (reader, please note, nothing is ever done tomorrow; things are only done right now), I recognized the power of now and felt excited. That was the day I realized what a powerful effect movement has on how you feel and, in a very short time, how you look, too. **That's how I identified the pillar of Movement.**

Night buses

I came to London in my early twenties, with fifty dollars and no plan. I look back on it now and wonder what the hell I was thinking. As we were landing, I remember turning to the person sitting next to me on the plane and asking her where I should stay. I genuinely had no idea what I was doing and, sure enough, within about two weeks, I was homeless.

I probably could have asked for help, but I was too proud. I was sleeping on night buses and eating food out of the bins outside Starbucks. I bought a suit and a pair of shoes from a charity shop (the shoes wore out within about a week, I resorted to patching them up with cardboard) and I managed to get myself a job at Harrods. I lived a double life for about eight weeks; I was working in one of the fanciest department stores on earth during the day, while sleeping rough at night.

That was my rock bottom. Some people have had worse rock bottoms and other people never get as low as being homeless. Experiencing that low was actually quite liberating. My choices were very clear-cut — I either survived or I didn't, I ate or went hungry. I chose to let nothing get in the way of my survival. I was able to use that positive mentality and it has stuck with me ever since. Rather than complaining, or sitting and wallowing, I was determined to succeed. It is that positivity which has made all the difference. **That's how I identified the pillar of Mindset.**

Tired of being tired

In my early thirties, I was working unhealthy hours as a personal trainer. I was constantly exhausted. If anyone ever asked me how I was, my default reponse was 'I'm tired'. I said that so many times that it started to define me. I was a tired person. My friend noticed this and said I needed to sort it out because I was going against the advice I gave my clients (that's why I always have compassion for people, because it's so easy for these unhealthy behaviours to sneak up on us without us even realizing it). I had become a 'very tired person' because (a) I wasn't sleeping, and (b) I'd convinced myself of it by repeating it over and over again. So I stopped telling people I was tired and I started really making a commitment to sleep. It was way more difficult than I had ever imagined. Not sleeping had become an addiction. Solving this lack of sleep was not just a question of going to bed earlier, I needed to change my behavioural patterns and my mindset, and it took some work. I experienced that terror of not being able to sleep. I used to stay up until I was exhausted, just so I didn't have to experience that 'I can't sleep' feeling. Over time, I worked at it. I researched and read and I started to learn new rituals, which got my body and mind ready to sleep. It improved everything. It improved my productivity, my happiness, my physical wellbeing, my relationships and it led to better choices, both at work and at home. It transformed how I felt physically and mentally. **That's how I identified the pillar of Sleep.**

MINDSET

Why is mindset a pillar of health?

Mindset is such an under-appreciated and under-acknowledged aspect of wellness. How do you get your body into shape? You exercise. How do you ensure physical transformation? You do it consistently, diligently, intelligently — and you stick to it. It's the same with mental health. I firmly believe that, just as we can use nutrition and exercise to help prevent poor physical health, we can take manageable steps to get our minds in the best possible shape, with the goal of living a long, happy, healthy life.

There's a lot of talk these days about mindfulness, but it's not just about doing yoga or downloading meditation apps (although there are some very good apps available, which I love). It is so much more than that. Yoga and meditation are simply gateways to learning the skills you need to attain mastery of your thoughts. Both will help you achieve optimum mental wellness, but the skills then need to be incorporated into your daily life, not just for the hour at yoga class or the 10 minutes spent meditating. For mindfulness to be effective, it needs to become part of the fabric of your life.

My wife, Christiane, made me realize the importance of mindset. When I first met Chrissy, I couldn't believe someone could truly be so happy. I was constantly scratching at the surface to see what was underneath. Finally, I realized that she was a genuinely positive and happy person, and once I'd seen that it was possible for Christiane (someone that I loved and trusted), I realized that it was possible for me, too. Because of how my mind works, I started to analyze her ability to always be positive, and I realized that we can teach ourselves to feel this way. Just like physical exercise, we should exercise our minds, too — they are as important as each other.

'Any change that happens in the body happens in the mind first.'

What does 'mindset' really mean?

Mindset to me means the mastery of your thoughts. There is a phenomenon that I often used to experience where I'd get a sudden feeling of dread or disappointment in the pit of my stomach, which would then hang over me for the rest of the day, week or sometimes even the month. I have learnt to actively stop this happening by investigating the feelings further before they take over my entire being and cause unnecessary stress. I pause and ask myself, 'Why am I feeling this way?' And then I search back through my mind and thoughts to work out what triggered it. I have come to understand that this sudden multitude of low feelings is caused by a negative situation, thought or memory that can usually be easily dealt with once you recognize it. Had I been aware of it at the time, I could have immediately addressed it, rationalized it, resolved it or, at the very least, made a conscious decision to either let it go or deal with it, rather than ending up with a constant hum at the back of my mind, dictating how I feel. Mindset is the process of investigating our negative feelings and learning to focus on positive thoughts. Allow your mindset to help master your thoughts.

What is the perfect body?

The perfect body is one that you feel happy and healthy in. There are plenty of people in the public eye who, despite having a low body-fat percentage and posting endless enviable 'selfies' online, are, in fact, constantly miserable. You can't have a 'perfect' body if you don't have a healthy mind. One of our Bodyism mantras is, 'Any change that happens in your body must happen in your mind first.' The key word here is 'first'. What you choose to eat, how often you move your body and the amount of rest you give yourself are determined by your thoughts. So your commitment to being healthy comes from how much you love and accept yourself.

Too many people are completely obsessed with how they look. They allow it to consume every aspect of their lives, which is far from healthy. There's often a 'when' mentality: when I am skinnier/more toned/have a flatter stomach — then I'll be happy. I've worked with well-known supermodels and actors for many years and I can absolutely promise you that the validation they are searching for (that we are all searching for) from other people will never be enough. It doesn't matter what you're seeking, be it a compliment from a friend or boyfriend, appearing on the cover of a magazine or winning an award for being 'the world's most beautiful', I guarantee you, it will never be enough.

We all suffer the same insecurities, self-doubt and fear of 'lacking'. It takes a huge amount of strength and self-discipline to get yourself off the misery train to crazy town. You need to value yourself beyond your weight or body-fat percentage. You need to value yourself for your kindness, talent, ideas and integrity, and only then will you begin to see a shift in your life as you finally start to experience 'it' — happiness. That elusive 'when' will finally become 'now'. With the right mindset, you can embrace the power of now. The perfect body is more about feeling mentally positive than anything else.

What are affirmations?

Affirmations are simply positive statements that define you as you want to be. Affirmations help make our goals feel real. If you look back through history, the words we speak have always been considered powerful. In every era and culture, when people want to find strength, they speak to a higher power — whether it's God, Buddha, Allah, Simon Cowell, whoever. To say something out loud is powerful. Choose your words wisely and use them kindly. The universe will listen to what you are saying; I truly believe that.

Chrissy and I have learnt from people far wiser than ourselves that the way you frame affirmations is really important. We phrase them as if the things we want are already in existence and we are already grateful for them. When you're grateful, it means something good has happened in your life, so simply to feel gratitude is one of the most positive and powerful states of being. You might say: 'Thank you for my healthy body.' You may not in fact have reached optimum health just yet, but by speaking of it as if it is already in existence, with no question or room for failure, makes it feel so much more achievable.

Here are some other examples you might try:

'Thank you for my happy life.'
'Thank you for my wonderful partner.'
'Thank you for my comfortable home.'
'Thank you for my nutritious food.'
'Thank you for my gold tooth.' (Okay, that one's a joke.)

Whatever it is that you are committed to bringing into your life, speak of it as if it has already happened, as if you are already grateful for it, and then imagine how it would feel to actually have it in your life. I've come to realize the power of affirmations and I've experienced the incredible effects of using them.

There is a lot of cynicism around affirmations. Those who doubt their power are the ones that aren't getting it. I think this is because people would rather be 'right' than happy. Let me explain.

Take, for example, a person who says, 'Everyone will screw you over.' With a strong negative view like this, they will probably find themselves drawn towards people that will screw them over, or they may create a situation where they are receiving poor treatment so they can be proved right about what they so firmly believe and have told themselves over and over again. Whatever it might be, the more you say it, the more 'right' you will be about it.

How can we make our minds positive?

I often tell my clients about a Cherokee legend called the 'Two Wolves', which clearly demonstrates the mastery we can achieve over our minds.

An elder Cherokee is teaching his grandson about life. 'A fight is going on inside me,' he says to the boy. 'It is a terrible fight and it is between two wolves. One is evil — he is anger, envy, sorrow, regret, greed, arrogance, self-pity, guilt, resentment, inferiority, lies, false pride, superiority and ego.' He continued, 'The other is good — he is joy, peace, love, hope, serenity, humility, kindness, benevolence, empathy, generosity, truth and compassion. The same fight is going on inside you   and inside every other person, too.'

The grandson thinks about it for a minute and then asks his grandfather, 'Which wolf will win?'

The old Cherokee simply replies, 'The one you feed.'

Our thoughts can be our own worst enemy, if we let them. Think about the negative stories you might be running in your mind. Many people believe they don't deserve a happy, healthy life. I can tell you right now, that is not true. You may tell yourself that you are 'not good enough', 'too stupid', 'too ugly' or any number of other things that don't serve you and are totally untrue. These are just unhelpful thoughts and don't have any purpose other than to reinforce habits that aren't constructive in any way at all. You've got to let all this stuff go because indulging in self-pity does not get you anywhere. Instead, you have the power to change the story you are running in your head. Once you are aware of it, you can then actively let the negative messages go.

A client of mine used to think, 'In order to be seen to be working hard, I have to be seen to be stressed and unhappy. I can't show any joy because then it looks like I'm not doing my job.' During our training sessions, I started to notice this. I asked her if she liked her job and she said she really did. I suggested to her that people would still think she is a hard

worker even if she smiled. She very quickly became aware of the negative story running in her head and from then on her general level of happiness increased, as did her productivity at work.

Similarly, I was at a party, chatting with a friend who works in the music industry. He wanted to talk to someone that he really admired, but couldn't pluck up the courage. I asked him why he wouldn't just go and introduce himself, especially since meeting this guy had the potential to improve his career. His response was, 'I'm just shy.'

I asked him, 'What makes you shy? Is there a shy gene? A shy cell? A shy hormone?'

For the first time, he actually stopped and thought about it, and eventually he said, 'No, there isn't a reason, maybe I'm not shy, it's just something I've been telling myself.'

That's a very powerful example of someone running a story in their head that has created a false construct of how things 'are'. You have the power to change your story, so make it a positive one. You can invent whatever you like about yourself. Tell yourself you are confident, you are loving and that you are capable of doing incredible things in this world. Change your story to that. Why not?

We all construct stories about ourselves in lots of different ways. It's not easy to step out of your internal comfort zone and really address these negative habits, but it is possible and can totally transform the way you experience the world. If you were overweight, you would probably look at your lifestyle and ask yourself, 'What am I eating?' or, 'How much am I exercising?' and then make changes. So, if you are emotionally unhappy, then why wouldn't you ask yourself: 'What do I generally think about?' or, 'What am I often preoccupied with?' or, 'What do I devote my mental energy to?' In other words, 'Which wolf do I feed?' (Whichever wolf you choose to feed, try to make it gluten free!)

How can I be more positive?

Most of what we worry about and the things that make us anxious, upset, stressed and miserable aren't actually happening and never will. The philosopher Michel de Montaigne said it best: 'My life has been full of terrible misfortunes most of which never happened.'

So let your worries go, because — remember — most of them will never happen. No more stressing about something at work, or a judgemental look that someone gave you (they're probably holding in a fart after eating a crappy lunch), or what someone else is thinking about you. It's important to know that everyone is just as self-obsessed as you are and they're probably not thinking about you at all. So, rather than getting caught up in negative thoughts, focus on the here and now.

Often, when I am stressed or anxious, I will do the following self-reflection exercise to remind myself of what I am grateful for in that very moment. So I might say, 'Right now, in this very moment, I am safe and warm, I am fed and I am okay. In this very moment. That is everything I've got.'

This exercise has saved me in the past because being present in that moment has empowered me to make strong decisions and choices, and has helped me navigate some very troubled times.

If, in that same moment, you are feeling sad or low, don't resist it, just accept it and let it pass like a cloud over a blue sky.

How can I break a habit?

I have been working for 20 years with clients who are 'giving up a habit', such as smoking or drinking. Often they've been working with a hypnotist or some form of 'guru', which never works because the only person that can put an end to your bad habits is you. There is no person or pill or magic spell that can change your life — it's you who can change your life. The power lies within you.

I fall very easily into habits and so I really do understand where people are coming from. I regularly slip back into bad habits before I even know it.

Here is an example of one of my (admittedly very lame) addictions...

For years, I would take a big slice of gluten-free bread, add loads of butter and then lather on this hazelnut spread. I ate it every night before bed and that was my 'thing'. It got to the point where I was in a complete cycle of addiction; I couldn't not have it. I always felt gross the next day — I had a constant food hangover. I used to hear this voice in my head (the gluttonous voice of stupidity) which would say, 'I really feel like it,' before starting to justify it even more with, 'I need it,' and, 'One more night makes no difference,' and, 'This is the last time.' It was probably more than three months before I ate it for the 'last' time. I could have gone on like that for the rest of my life.

This is possibly the nerdiest story of addiction ever told and I'm almost embarrassed that I don't have a heavier story to share, but it doesn't matter what the addiction is; it's the same thing, the same voices justifying it. It doesn't have to be alcohol or drugs to make you an addict.

So, finally, I had to admit to myself, 'I am addicted. My drug of choice is gluten-free bread and hazelnut spread.' (And, yes, I see the humour in this addiction story!) It's frightening how easily you can talk yourself into things. That voice in my head is very, very persuasive and so I had to say, 'I have got to stop.' I said no to the temptation, I shut the cupboard door and I held tight. I had a rubbish night or two, but I got through it.

Remember, it's not just the substance you get addicted to — it's the ritual. For me, it was the motion of putting the bread in the toaster, layering on the butter, lathering on the spread. It's the same for those who crave a glass of wine at night. The answer is to swap it for a healthy habit that fulfils the same function. Find a healthy ritual that fills the void. Instead of pouring yourself a glass of wine, treat yourself to five minutes of yoga or relaxing breathing, a warm bath or a cup of tea. Does that sound less satisfying? Maybe. Will it change your life? Definitely. Go for a walk, listen to some music. Find a healthy replacement for the bad habit.

There is no secret technique to doing this. If there were, then a lot more people would be free from their bad habits and significantly fewer people would be obese, unhealthy and unhappy. There is no shame in being an addict. So many of us (me included) have that personality trait, DNA or chemical make up, but you just need to recognize that a particular habit is making you miserable and that it needs to stop. Ask yourself, 'Why do I want to break my habit?' If you have a strong enough 'why', then it will carry you through the challenge of breaking any bad habit that might otherwise be too difficult.

One of the most difficult habits to break is late-night eating. I asked naturopath Rhaya Jordan for her five ways to break that habit, and here is what she advised:

1. Wear yourself out. Most of us are too sedentary in the day (sitting at our desks, sitting for our commute and sitting some more for lunch). So, if you can, try to use up your physical energy within your day — even if that means getting up 30 minutes earlier to walk to the next bus stop, or going on a quick walk during your lunch break or after dinner. Tire yourself out so you actually want to go to bed at a sensible hour.

2. Fuel up. So many people under-eat during the day and then make up for it at night. Think through your schedule logically. In the morning, you will need to power yourself up with enough energy for the day, so have a wonderful, nourishing breakfast (take inspiration from the Breakfast chapter, see pages 94–117). Then, rather than underfeeding yourself (and dragging your metabolism down with you), eat when you are hungry during the day, so that at night (after a nourishing dinner) you can let your body and mind wind down rather than stressing it out with unnecessary late grazing.

3. Create a rest routine. Sleep is nature's gift, so be thankful for it! Come up with rituals that help you wind down, as these will make you way happier (and healthier) than late-night snacking. Light a relaxing candle (remembering to blow it out before you go to sleep), keep your bed looking comfy (think big squashy pillows and a beautiful soft throw), drink a cup of herbal tea or read a good book in bed. Reserve your bedroom just for sleep or sex, and take any stress out of there. When you start looking forward to bed, the temptation to eat might loosen its grip.

4. Say it straight. When your inner grazer starts tempting you into the kitchen, remind yourself that sleep deprivation is a huge factor in weight gain. It makes you put on weight, thickens your waist and is just as fattening as alcohol. Be strict with yourself.

5. Be a night gazer (not a night grazer). The end of the day is a wonderful time to reassess your goals. Write them down, watch a movie that gets you thinking or chat to someone you care about. Switch off the TV food shows, which do nothing but wake up your dangerous grazer, and do something that you'll be proud of in the morning.

How do you get your partner to buy into a healthy mindset when you are already there?

The truth is you can't. The minute you try to 'fix' someone, it's inevitably going to make them feel broken. But you can encourage them subtly with small changes. So, if you are doing the food shopping or the cooking, then make sure you invite your partner to eat nourishing meals with you. And rather than saying, 'You need to go to the gym,' suggest going for a walk together. Make it a fun thing that you do together.

Change comes through inspiration, by being shown how good something can make you feel. No one ever had their mind changed by being told they were not good enough; they have to realize the benefits of change for themselves. Often, people might be reluctant because their self-esteem is low, in which case telling them they are lazy or fat, or that they need to do it, can be counter-productive. You have to live your own life, make those changes for yourself, and hopefully your partner will be inspired, encouraged, motivated and supported enough to do it with you.

How does my physical health affect my mental health?

I see the incredible effects of exercise every day in people who walk through the Bodyism doors. Shy, introverted people enter with a general fog of unhappiness surrounding them, but then they get their bodies moving and blood pumping and they transform, not just physically, but also (and more importantly) mentally. They begin to smile more, they start to glow, and they generally look and feel more confident and happy.

Moving your body can only make you feel better, no two ways about it. It changes you on a hormonal and physical level. You don't have to go mad on a treadmill (in fact, you shouldn't), you can just go for a walk or do some yoga, but whatever it is, simply moving your body will help you hit a natural high.

When you are feeling stressed, angry or anxious, rather than stewing over it, go for a walk and get your body moving. I remember once, when I was in a really dark place and things weren't going well, I rang Chrissy and she said to me, 'Go for a surf, just for me.' I thought it was a ridiculous suggestion — we had so much to sort out and I had people to ring and emails to send — but I listened to her. I went for a surf and, I promise you, my entire life transformed. Everything that seemed insurmountable suddenly became solvable. All the complications became simple. It transported me to a point where I could see a way out. So I always say, if you are stressed or angry and don't know what to do, move your body and then reassess; it could make the world of difference in realizing what you need to do.

What does it mean to be kind to yourself?

One of the driving philosophies of Bodyism is 'Be kind to yourself'. We believe in this phrase so much that we had it carved in stone at the front of Bodyism, London.

What does this mean? Being kind to yourself means understanding that you deserve a happy, healthy life. Recognizing that you are good enough, are worth listening to and are worth loving. I say this is because so many people feel worthless, undeserving and unlovable — but you are none of those things. I don't know everything, but I know this for sure. Once you recognize that, all the choices you make become easy. The pursuit of health stops being a battle and becomes a joyful way of life that elevates your experience of the world. Let this philosophy guide you through every section of this book and every aspect of your life. As you work through the four pillars of health, make being kind to yourself your guiding principle.

So how do you do this? By choosing foods that make you feel good; by choosing to think powerful, positive thoughts; by choosing to surround yourself with people who support, encourage and empower you. Remind yourself that you deserve a long, happy and healthy life, reaffirm your strengths and change that negative inner conversation to a positive one. Recite positive affirmations to yourself, such as, 'I am unstoppable', 'I am a good friend' and 'I am a powerful person', and really believe them — because, whichever story you tell yourself, will eventually be the one that comes true. Make it real and live your happily ever after, not just your 'generally-unsatisfied-about-my-body-weight' ever after. No fairytale ever ended that way.

NUTRITION

'Diets do not work.'

Why is nutrition a pillar of health?

Many people still haven't made the connection between what they eat and how they feel. They don't understand that nutrition is one of the four pillars of health. My goal in writing this chapter is to give you a deeper understanding of the effect food has on how you look, how you feel and even who you are. I also want you to be able to show this to those you love so that you can inspire change in them, too. What people eat today will not only affect their health immediately, but will have long-term effects, too.

Over the years, I've been asked questions such as, 'What is better to have in my water — lemon or lime?' and, 'Which berry is best?' and, 'What is the exact amount of protein I should be consuming each day?' But my advice is please don't worry about those kinds of small details, because they just act as a distraction from what you really need to be asking. You need to be asking the bigger and more powerful questions which will genuinely make a positive impact. Questions like, 'How am I feeling now, after eating that?' and, 'What am I going to do differently next time?' The answers are all within ourselves. This chapter will shine a light on how to ask the right questions.

To help you find the answers, I asked Rhaya Jordan, a highly respected naturopath who we work with here at Bodyism, to share her expertise. I hope her knowledge inspires you and equips you with a new-found understanding and passion for nutrition.

What does healthy eating mean?

Often, people with the best intentions do all the wrong things. I remember clients coming into Bodyism in the early days, saying, 'My cholesterol is high; I need to stop eating whole eggs and I can't have oily fish,' and we would try to very gently show them the research that disproves that whole way of thinking. All the things I've been saying at Bodyism for over 15 years are finally becoming mainstream and widely accepted. The sad thing is that millions of people have died or suffered in the meantime, thinking they were doing the 'right' thing. So it's time we knew which guidelines are truly healthy and what we are being told is, in fact, good for our health.

I don't know about you, but I'm so disillusioned and exhausted with all the different advice and diets out there. Which ones and who should you trust? It's enough to drive even the most logical person insane.

Health no longer smells like lentils. It has become so much sexier and more superficial over the past few years and therefore it's harder to navigate. I remember, 30 years ago, you'd go into a health-food store and the person working there would be wearing a jumper made out of leaves, with bloodshot, sleepy eyes and they'd look like they had wandered out of a commune — it was scary. I used to ask my mum, 'Why are all the health-food people weird? And why do they look so sick?'

Health isn't weird anymore. Now it's mainstream, slick and (for lack of a better word) 'cool'. Wellness has become a very powerful industry, which can be a hugely positive thing if people are listening to the right messages, but when they are being sold something damaging, it can also be very scary and dangerous for their health. It's only recently that people have started to see through some of these health bloggers who have no life experience or professional qualifications — and who are ruining this wonderful industry. Please be aware of people out there who are dressing up their eating disorders with a green juice; the truth is that they are just finding a different and more sophisticated way of saying

'Please be obsessed with your food', and it is giving others an excuse to justify such obsessions. This new flowery language of food 'empowerment' is often driven by nothing but shame and guilt. Constantly asking yourself, 'What am I going to eat?' or 'Did I eat too much?' or 'Is it free from (insert almost everything here)?' is far worse than any diet. It's an eating disorder and it's got a name — it's called orthorexia.

For example, there's an Instagram user who recommends eating 30 bananas per day. This isn't something I've made up; it's a real person who has thousands of followers and is ruining people's lives every day. Anyone who follows that person, or other similar accounts, and takes their advice to eat nothing but fruit is obviously stupid and has zero understanding of human biology. Our bodies just don't work like that.

Here I am, saying it again: the only thing that works is balance. The minute you begin to weigh your food, count your calories or beat yourself up for going out for dinner, it's over. You are on a countdown to yet another unsuccessful 'diet'.

I wish I could provide you with 'healthy eating' rules, but they just don't work because rules are made to be broken and, more importantly, the human body does not respond well to rules. We are more complicated than that. There is only one rule to remember: be kind to yourself. It should drive every single choice you make. Beyond that, what works for one person won't work for another. So, rather than going on a restrictive banana diet, which is not good for you and will only plague you with shame and guilt, all you need to do is tune into your body and find foods which work for you. Your body will soon thank you for it and return to its natural state of 'vibrant aliveness'.

How does mindset affect nutrition?

The Bodyism food philosophy isn't just about what you eat, it's also very much about how you think. How you think drives what you eat and how you feel. It's all interconnected, and the four pillars are each equally important.

The energy you put into your food is almost as important as *what* you are eating. If you have an unhealthy attitude towards food, return to the affirmations I mentioned in the Mindset chapter (see pages 12–23). Affirmations really help with that 'mental arm-wrestle' that so many people are struggling with. If I'm at home and am bored, I tend to become 'psychologically starving' and that's when it's impossible to listen to my body. But, rather than going straight to the fridge, take a moment and pause. Remind yourself of your affirmations: 'I am eating to nourish myself'; 'I am grateful for this food'. That moment of reminding yourself to 'be kind' will make all the difference.

In the past, my attitude towards food has been unhealthy. I grew up hungry, because we never had enough food, so even once I'd pulled my life together and I knew where my next meal was coming from, I still had that frightened eight-year-old inside me, telling me to eat everything I could. Here I was, pioneering an entirely new approach to food, health and wellness, and yet I was still eating obsessively. I would eat everything in my path until I was totally full. When I finally recognized the underlying beliefs that were driving my behaviour and telling me I had to eat like that, I was able to acknowledge that it wasn't working for me, and only then did it stop. It helped me kick that obsessive behaviour, and the unfounded belief that food was scarce. Once I became aware of it, I was able to change it.

When you become aware of negative beliefs which drive negative behaviours, make a conscious effort to replace them with more positive beliefs, and it will significantly change the way you eat and the foods you choose.

When does healthy become unhealthy?

Chrissy and Nathalie (a Bodyism inspiration and a total hero!) really taught me the importance of balance. I used to overeat (on 'healthy' foods) and feel constantly bloated and uncomfortable. I lived on nothing but green vegetables, fish and meat; I would feel guilty if I had any sort of carbs and I was always underperforming in everything I did. I'd live in a cycle of restriction and bingeing on 'cheat meals' (see page 41). Mentally, I'm strong, so I would ignore how tired I felt. I got used to being dizzy: when I trained, in meetings and just in general. On the outside, I looked fit and well and was eating a very 'healthy' diet. I look back on it and can now recognize that I was being totally restrictive and I was 'gassed out'.

After being around Chrissy and Nat, they told me to start bringing abundance into my diet, eat lots of colours, beans, brown rice, sweet potatoes and fruit, and to have a more varied diet. So I did the Bodyism Two-week Blueprint (see pages 80–91), stopped eating my 'cheat meal' on the weekend and that obsessive behaviour went away very quickly. I stopped beating myself up and took a leap of faith, and I started to enjoy eating from a more varied diet. That shame and guilt disappeared and I began to really tune in to how my body felt. When I finally started to eat a bit of everything, I began to 'feel' energized, rather than simply 'acting' it. And now I look better than I've ever looked and I've never felt happier and healthier.

Always remember that the middle ground is the safest, healthiest and happiest place to be — it's fun here in the middle. It's the people on the edges who are angry, boring and unhealthy.

Rhaya Jordan: Feeling relaxed and flexible (mentally) are nice hallmarks of being healthy. When you feel angry at yourself for eating something 'unhealthy', or if you can't concentrate on anything but your body or food, then that is stressful and not healthy. Here is the key, base your self-worth on the deep respect you have for yourself rather than what you see on the scales. If seeing that you've put on an extra pound ruins your day, you need to back off a bit and get some perspective. You deserve to be well — that's true health.

Why don't diets work?

Diets are based on denial. If I tell you not to think of the Eiffel Tower, it will be the first thing that comes into your mind. Similarly, if I say not to eat cake, most people reading this won't be able to stop thinking about it until the stupid diet they are on finally finishes and they can eat all of the cake — yes, all of it. This phenomenon can be summed up in one phrase: 'What you resist, persists.' So, rather than fighting against your cravings and making it a battle, simply let it go.

What does this mean? I hear you ask. The minute you make it a battle, there is only ever going to be one winner and it won't be you. When you can relax, stop fighting and understand that you deserve to be happy and healthy, all of these battles become choices and the choices become easy. The key is not focusing on and thinking about what you can't have, and instead focusing on what you can have. So often, health is focused on giving things up, when actually it should be about enjoying amazing food which improves how you feel — and once you've experienced that, there's no going back. You might slip off the wagon, but, 'Nothing tastes as good as *healthy* feels.' (Consider me the Kate Moss of wellness!)

So, if you're choosing foods that work for you, make you feel good and taste delicious, are you on a diet? Or are you just living a happier, healthier, more intelligent life? Instead of going on a diet, how about you decide to finally be kind to yourself and completely change your life?

When I say, 'Be kind to yourself,' it's more than just a slogan or a cliché, because what I mean is that you should let go of shame and guilt. Understand that your past doesn't equal your future; if you have failed before, use it as a lesson. Failure is feedback. Accept yourself, so that you can create a powerful platform from which to move forward towards a happier, healthier you.

You still thinking about the Eiffel Tower? Now you are. That's why diets don't work.

Rhaya Jordan: Nutrition is a marathon, not a sprint. One of the best ways to look after your overall health is to change your behaviour surrounding food, rather than signing up to another diet. Fundamentally, if you want to embark on real, deep change, you have to work with your body.

Ask yourself, 'What food do I enjoy?' 'What time of day am I hungry?' 'Does gluten/dairy/sugar make me irritable or sleepy, or fill me with energy?'

Everyone is different and lots of these differences will be genetic, while some of them will be because of your gut microbiome (the natural bacteria in your digestive system). If you eat when you're hungry and stop when you're not, eat whole foods you enjoy and trust your body, you will get there.

Sometimes, people will need to do a 'sprint' — maybe before a holiday in the sun or a big event — and, if that's the case, then try the Bodyism Two-week Blueprint (see pages 88–91), which cuts out the main irritants for a fortnight and is a great way to refresh your system and work out what your gut likes and dislikes. But, if you eat poorly, then restrict, and then go back to eating poorly again, those extremes will cause more damage. The middle, balanced path is what's going to change your life forever.

What should I eat for breakfast?

What you have for breakfast will set up your body, psychology and hormonal profile for the rest of the day. It will also determine what you crave throughout the day. So, if you start your day with sugar, you will find yourself on an all-day sugar rollercoaster. This is where the importance of sleep comes in (the final pillar, see pages 74–87), because if you don't have a good night's sleep, you're more likely to crave a quick sugar fix the next morning (more on this later).

As I've said from the off, we are all different, so there is no hard-and-fast rule for everyone. I am what's called a 'fast oxidizer', which means (put simply) that I digest food very quickly. So, when I eat porridge/oatmeal for breakfast, it very quickly spikes my blood sugar levels and then I also crash pretty quickly. Chrissy, on the other hand, is a slow oxidizer. She can eat pasta, porridge or potatoes, and they're digested slowly and don't give her a sugar spike. She doesn't get the mood swings that I do, and her blood sugar levels don't dip and dive like mine. On the flip side, I can eat butter, eggs, avocado and steak all in one go and, because I digest food so quickly, I don't end up feeling heavy; in fact, I feel energized — whereas a slow oxidizer would find that difficult for their body to deal with. It's why the Bodyism coffee (Americano blended with coconut oil and butter) works well for me, but is too heavy for some people. So, it's all about testing things out to find the breakfast for you.

As a general rule of thumb, it is really important to start the day with some protein. You need it to nourish yourself and keep you feeling full and energized throughout the morning. Day to day, it's all about tuning in to your body. One morning, you may crave lots of carbohydrates and energy, and you will feel really great from eating that; then, on other mornings, you might feel more like a big helping of protein. Some mornings I wake up and crave eggs, avocado and spinach cooked in butter, while other mornings I just fancy a breakfast salad. Two years ago, if you had suggested the latter to me for breakfast, I would have turned on my heel and stormed out. Now, I have tuned in to my body.

It takes a while to really understand what it means to 'tune in' to your body, so while you are learning, I'll remind you of what doesn't work, and that is sugary breakfast cereals. These are virtually devoid of any nutritional value at all, and a bowl for breakfast will make your blood sugar spike and have you craving sugar for the rest of the day. If you're reading this thinking that you like your breakfast cereal, the reality is that you don't — it's just that you're addicted to the sugar hit. Try giving it up and having something different, such as half an avocado sliced up on oatcakes, or some oats, nuts and seeds soaked in rice milk. For those thinking, 'Are you crazy?' — just try it; you might love it! It's so much better for you to eat a beautiful creamy avocado or crunchy oatcakes than a bowl of sugar- and salt-filled processed cereal. Not to mention that ditching the toast and cereal sets you well on your way to a flat, bloat-free stomach. Remember the quote at the start of the book: 'Be open to everything, to all possibilities, listen and be curious.'

Rhaya Jordan: Your first meal of the day should set you up for everything that follows, so make sure your breakfast is of high quality. An almond croissant to start your day will only send you spinning off on that sugar rollercoaster and you'll feel exhausted by lunchtime. There is so much new information coming out about our microbiome and how it affects the way we digest food. There are lots of different theories in terms of why we might find different combinations work well for us individually.

Of course, tuning in to your body has to be balanced with the demands of modern life. If you don't feel hungry till mid-morning, then just be prepared and, instead of going to your local convenience store and picking up something highly processed, spend 10 minutes the night before preparing your bowl of porridge (Three-Grain Porridge, see page 100), or keep some blueberries and almonds at work to enjoy when you are finally ready to eat. Try things out, find a pattern that fits your body and the end result will be much better. Appetite changes and varies, so tuning in to your body is the only answer. Intuitive eating is the Holy Grail.

Top Tip Start your day with food before your coffee (even if the food is a smoothie). Enjoy your coffee, but find balance and don't use it to replace breakfast (or to drive yourself when you're exhausted). The biggest problem with coffee is how easy it is to use it as a distraction from the real problem. If your coffee habit is to make up for a lack of sleep and rest, then listen to your body and go to bed earlier instead of having a third or fourth cup.

What should I eat for breakfast if I have no time in the mornings?

1. **Smoothies.** Before you go to bed, put all of your whole ingredients in the blender and then all you need to do in the morning is pour in the liquid and blend it up. That takes less than five minutes. See pages 216–219 for some great recipes.

2. **Jar prep.** Pay yourself respect and prepare. It takes just five minutes before you go to bed to fill a jar with our Simply Granola (see page 102), ready to add milk to once you get to work, or make a Bircher Muesli (see page 101), which you can leave overnight in the fridge and then throw in your bag and eat on the bus.

3. **On-the-go.** Pots of boiled eggs and spinach can be bought in most food stores nowadays and, although less interesting than something home-made, they are ideal if you are struggling for time, and will give you what you need to start the day off right.

4. **Go fish!** There's a great British tradition of eating fish for breakfast. Pick up some sardines, kippers and smoked haddock or even some prawns/shrimp, if you can stomach it! Seafood is high in protein and a great option if you don't feel like eggs.

5. **Fruit 'n' nut.** If you are really stuck for time, then just grab yourself a small punnet of berries and some almonds — you can find those anywhere!

Rhaya Jordan: A smoothie is such a fast, easy, nutrient-packed meal. If you are rushing, it's a top choice, because the fact the food has been blended means it will be easier to digest and more soothing for your stressed-out digestive system. Please remember that smoothies you make at home are in a different league to the smoothies from a supermarket, which are normally higher in sugar than a fizzy drink. Smoothies in a supermarket shouldn't be called smoothies; they should be renamed liquid lollies. Comparing home-made and shop-bought smoothies is like comparing a Michelin-star noodle dish to a cup of instant noodles.

What should I eat when I'm out?

Enjoy your meal out and don't amplify the damage or ruin it with feelings of shame and guilt. When choosing what to eat, think about what you will genuinely enjoy and what makes you feel happy, not just in the short term, but for the rest of the day or evening. So, yes, it might bring you a sort of 'pleasure' to have the bread basket and then a big plate of pasta and a chocolate cake, but if it will make you feel miserable, lethargic and bloated soon after, then maybe reassess which dishes will genuinely make you feel amazing. If you are somewhere that sells delicious fresh produce, like wild fish with seasonal vegetables, give it a go, as I guarantee you will feel fantastic after eating it (unless you're allergic to fish, of course). The trick is not to think about what you 'can't' have, but to focus on all the other amazing things that you can have.

How can I minimize damage from alcohol?

No one 'has' to drink. Anyone who says they have to drink because of their job, or for whatever reason, is kidding themselves, because it's just not true, and when clients tell me this, I simply don't buy it. You always have a choice. From a personal point of view, I choose not to drink alcohol, and yet, in spite of this, I still manage to live a full and happy life. Take responsibility for your own life and your own health. There are other people that can do it, so what's so different about you? Those people value their health, but they still enjoy themselves responsibly and have a great work-life balance. Remind yourself of your 'why' before you make a decision (as I said before, mine is to live a long, happy and healthy life) and let that influence you. If you really do want one drink, then — fine — do it, own it and move on from it. Remember, alcohol, by its nature, is a poison. Just the words and language used to describe it prove that: 'getting drunk', 'getting wasted', 'getting smashed', 'getting written off'. None of those are positive. 'I'm going to go out and get uplifted,' said no one, ever.

Rhaya Jordan: If you are going out somewhere to eat, go out and enjoy it! What makes the difference is your day-to-day intake, so a special one-off night out for dinner isn't something you should ever feel bad about. The French are a great inspiration, because they have the lowest obesity levels in the whole of Europe, despite the fact that they love cake. They enjoy food in small doses, lingering over their food, enjoying it mindfully and eating it slowly. Also, remind yourself that you can have beautiful, indulgent food whenever you want; so, rather than eating everything in sight, remind yourself that you can come back and enjoy food like this again. This mindset will stop you from bingeing and purging (cake will always be around, so there's no need to eat it all up every time you go out). Eating out only starts to be a problem when you do it most nights, and that is when you might want more guidance. If your goal is weight loss, lean heavily on vegetables and go for protein, as it tends to help you avoid extra hidden sugars. Salads are always a good option, as are soups.

Rhaya Jordan: Alcohol is a carbohydrate, a simple one, and it does a lot of damage to your gut, your brain and your liver. Most alcohol is sweetened with some form of sugar or syrup and, because our gut is trying to expel the alcohol as quickly as possible, the sugar in the cocktail or glass of wine is very quickly converted into fat. So, whether we like it or not, alcohol is fattening and, more importantly, is not good for you. You can't 'limit' the damage from alcohol, but what you can do is slow down the rate of absorption by having a meal with your glass of wine (or cocktail, if you must). You will feel the effect of the alcohol less quickly (so you won't say or sing things you regret), but don't forget you will still be consuming the same amount, just more slowly. If you do decide to drink, my 'tips' for alcohol are:

1. **Choose red wine.** It's the only alcohol that's associated with any good health outcomes. But still keep your intake low and try to stick to no more than two glasses of wine (and always consider it a treat rather than a necessity).

2. **Keep it clean.** The cocktail with the least amount of sugar is vodka and soda. That's a much wiser choice than eggnog! Remember what I said: the sugar from cocktails converts to fat very quickly.

3. **The one cocktail.** If you are desperate for a cocktail, go for a freshly made Bloody Mary, as the tomato juice will have some benefits — but please make sure it's not lined with sugar syrup.

4. **Green cocktails.** Some fancy bars are now offering green juices as a mixer for spirits. Obviously these are wonderful, minus the alcohol.

5. **Say, 'Cheers!'** Celebration and delight are incredibly powerful tonics; so, if you are going to raise a glass of Champagne, don't then stress yourself out with feelings of shame and guilt. Own it, trust yourself not to drink the whole bottle, enjoy the celebration and then move on.

What should I eat when I have no time to cook?

First of all, it's important to make time to eat. Every now and then you may not be able to, and I do get that, because it's the reality of life, but bear in mind that if you have time to scroll through Instagram, then you have time to eat. If you often end up eating on the go, you are not being kind to yourself and you need to change that habit. Eating is what makes us energized, strong and powerful, so respect yourself and make time for it.

It would be wonderful if we could all eat lightly steamed vegetables that we grew ourselves from organic seeds foraged on a trip to Peru which had been blessed by a monk. The reality is that most people's lives just aren't anything like this. Instead, you may have to grab whatever you've got to hand when you're at home or on the go, and that means making sure you create an environment which influences healthy habits and 'bulletproofs' your life from unhealthy options.

When you make dinner, it's a great idea to always make extra. That way, when you have 'no time to eat', you've got something ready to go from the night before.

On the weekend, I bake a big batch of chicken thighs with Italian herbs, or lemon and ginger, or the Bodyism rub (see The Only Rub You'll Ever Need on page 214). I'll enjoy a few thighs for dinner with brown rice and steamed greens, and then keep the rest in the fridge for a super-nourishing, delicious, high-protein snack whenever I fancy it throughout the week (it's also better than what you can find in most take-out shops).

If you haven't had time to make anything the night before, use your knowledge of whole, unprocessed foods. If you're out and about, rather than reaching for fast food, buy some whole 'real' foods: cold meats, hummus, nuts and vegetables. You can get all of these at most convenience stores.

Will carbs make me put on weight?

Just to be clear, and keeping it very simple, there are real carbs and there are trash carbs. Choose your carbs wisely.

REAL CARBS
Oats · Sweet potatoes · Broccoli · Squash · Parsnips · Swede/rutabaga · Brown rice · Quinoa · Rye · Barley · Spelt

TRASH CARBS
White flour · Sugar · White bread · White pasta · Shop-bought granola

Rhaya Jordan: Carbs won't necessarily make you put on weight. In fact, the Okinawans have the greatest proportion of centenarians in the world, and they tend to be lean and slender, despite the fact they eat a large amount of rice. If it was true that carbs were the 'demon', then none of the world's healthiest populations would eat them... but they all do.

So here is the problem: when we think of 'carbs', we think of refined, processed, rubbish carbs. Get rid of that image and instead choose beautiful wholegrains. Adding a portion of these grains into your meal can be really satisfying. As always, listen to your body. If you feel good after eating them, then you've found a really great way to make your body feel full and content (and you'll therefore snack less between meals). Of course, it comes back to that individuality again, because some people can eat porridge/oatmeal for breakfast and yet still feel hungry all day. In case you want to know the science, there's an enzyme in the body called 'amylase', which helps you break down carbohydrates. The more amylase you have (which is determined by genetics), the more easily you digest carbs.

Many people think if they cut out carbs, they will lose weight. This isn't a lifestyle goal; it's a 'quick fix' which can leave your overall health (and metabolism) the worse for wear. If you have a carbohydrate sensitivity, that is different, but if you want to look and feel good for the long term, remind yourself of balance: eat carbs, observe how you feel and alter portions accordingly.

Word of warning: bad carbs suit no one.

Is not eating sugar a trend?

Sugar can make you fat, sick and, to be frank, can even lead to an early, otherwise preventable death, so cutting back on sugar is definitely not a trend. Sugar converts to fat quicker than fat itself because it raises insulin levels, which causes fat storage. Studies show that 40 per cent of the sugar you eat is converted straight to fat (that's in a slim person). Sugar leaches vitamins from your body, and a body starved of vitamins is a hungry one. As I've always said, 'low-fat' food and drinks are packed with sugar, as they've substituted the fat for processed ingredients — so they may not contain fat, but they will still make you fat. Don't buy them.

So should you cut sugar out completely? It depends on who you are. Refined sugar can be a trigger food. It can give you a sugar rush and behaves like a drug. It gets very hard for people to keep their equilibrium. Some people (like me) will find sugar so addictive that one sliver of cake becomes 37.

I have to cut refined sugar out completely because I'm an addict. I'll convince myself that I really do need a chocolate cake and that I deserve it and it's fine, and then I'll eat it every day until, two months later, I end up in Las Vegas, lying in a pile of chocolate cake, wondering how I got there. So, I know not to start down that slippery slope.

Instead, I enjoy natural sugars from fruit, but I also know when I've had enough. I've learnt to listen to my body.

And what's the deal with all of these 'pretend' sugars? Be aware of the cool kids who pretend to be your friend, but aren't really, including coconut palm sugar, agave, brown rice syrup, maple syrup, honey and dates. In the same way that getting slapped in the face is marginally better than getting kicked in the head, they are not quite as terrible as refined sugar, but they still aren't ever going to be good for you. It's not a magic solution, so please don't think, 'I can have as much of this as I want.' They still affect your blood sugar levels, your hormonal profile and your weight. You may find maple syrup or other unrefined sugars don't hit you as hard as refined sugar, but if it is your drug, just steer clear.

It's also worth knowing that there are people in the wellbeing industry who are thought of as beacons of health, and yet produce and promote 'health snacks' that actually contain more sugar than a chocolate bar. Every now and then, a newspaper will run a scandalous story on it and a few people may become aware of the reality, but the vast majority will continue to buy these 'healthy' snacks under the mistaken notion that they are actually good for them. Can I remind you, just because they are wrapped in brown paper and labelled organic or gluten-free, it doesn't make them any more healthy or less fattening.

Rhaya Jordan: If sugar was rationed tomorrow and it wasn't in so many drinks as well as savoury food, then we could relax about a pudding or a bit of homemade cake. Back in the fifties, sugar wasn't an everyday staple — it was a treat. But the way the food industry works now is so back to front, and sugar finds its way into practically everything, distorting your brain signals and making you wander into an addictive relationship with it. I'm shocked by how much sugar is in processed foods — sauces, cereals, drinks, even cold meats! The list goes on and on, and it's all gone totally insane. In the same vein, we shouldn't go to the other extreme and feel guilty about eating fruit or a slice of cake from time to time. As always, the middle path is the healthy option.

Rhaya Jordan: Until you really start to nourish your digestion and care for your body, you might have no idea what your true personality or mood is. There are two main ways in which we tend to undermine our digestion:

1. **How we eat.** We are designed to digest food properly only when we are relaxed. Remember, we are mammals, and our four-legged friends would not sit down for a meal if a lion was around; they'd be getting out of the way. To put this in modern terms, eating 'on the run' is a disaster, because it makes us miss out a key stage of digestion called the 'cephalic' stage. If you have ever walked past delicious-smelling food and felt your mouth water, then you know what this stage is: it's when you release enzymes into saliva which help break down your food. When you miss this stage out, your food doesn't get broken down properly and you get more fermentation, bloating and gas. One of the key characteristics of people who live long, healthy lives is that they sit down to eat their meals. Chewing really well makes an enormous difference to your overall health — it could be the one thing that can transform your gut.

2. **What we eat.** Our gut is populated by trillions of bacteria that have a symbiotic relationship with our body. Justin and Erica Sonnenburg explain it perfectly: 'Our microbiome (the gut bacteria) contains 100 times more genes than our human genome, so in fact there is about 99 percent of associated genetic material that we have the potential to mould in ways that are beneficial to us.'

Our gut biome has an enormous impact on our overall wellness. Also, the microbiome determines how much weight you put on from the food you eat. Put simply, a group of bacteria called 'firmicutes' are associated with weight gain. They change the way your body absorbs your food, and they love refined carbohydrates (sugar), which means when you choose processed foods, you are creating the perfect environment for firmicutes to grow, which in turn encourages fat storage. On the other hand, the group of bacteria called 'bacteroidetes' help you metabolize food and have also been linked to reducing the risk of obesity, as well as illnesses like Crohn's disease and cancer. They love fibre, so choosing vegetables and fermented foods will help you get more bacteroidetes in your gut.

How does my gut affect my health?

We are suffering an unnecessary amount of gut problems in our modern world because people aren't nourishing their bodies and generally do not go to the toilet enough. We're friends now, so I can say it: you should do a poo every day. One of the biggest-selling pharmaceutical products is laxatives. This has got to stop. Last year, the US Food and Drug Administration warned that the side effects of laxatives include severe dehydration, kidney damage and swelling of the legs and feet. The other option is to eat more leafy green vegetables and fibrous foods. Surely, it's obvious that we need to think more long term about how to improve our gut health. The connection between your gut and your brain is so strong that even physicians have begun referring to the gut as your 'second brain'. It's where your 'gut instinct' comes from.

Do calories count?

No. On a psychological level, counting calories simply doesn't work because, as humans, we are just not designed to eat by numbers. The minute you bring that kind of thinking into the way you eat, you take all the joy out of it and it turns into a slippery slope of obsessive behaviour and control, which can lead to eating disorders.

What a lot of people don't know is that, not only does calorie counting not work, but it's often totally inaccurate. The calorie content of food changes constantly. To accurately work out the total number of calories that you get from a given food, you'd have to take into account a ridiculous amount of factors, including the following:

1. How boiling, steaming, baking or slow-cooking the food changes its structure and chemistry.

2. How much energy the body uses up by digesting the food.

3. The extent to which billions of bacteria in the gut help human digestion and, conversely, use calories during the process of digestion.

It will never be exact. Ever. So counting calories becomes a pointless losing battle.

It's such a futile and simplistic approach. For example, if you look at the calories in an avocado compared to a bag of sweets, there will be more in the avocado. That obviously doesn't mean you should reach for the candy instead, though, does it? The sugar in the sweets converts to fat, which is stored around your internal organs and your tummy, whereas the avocado contains essential fats, which can help speed up your metabolism and will keep you feeling fuller for longer.

When I started working as a personal trainer, I spent time working in one of the best gyms in Europe. They've got this incredible measurement system which works out how many calories you will burn throughout a day. Then they design an eating and exercise plan that puts you in calorie deficit. Sounds amazing, right? It's completely rubbish. Why, I hear you ask? Because real life gets in the way. On Tuesday, it might be 'Dennis's birthday' and you have to eat a cupcake, which throws out your entire day, or, on Wednesday, you might have to stay out late and you can't go to the gym. It's great if you're a billionaire and you don't have to 'live' life, or you don't have a partner, children, job or anything else like that. But, for most of us, that isn't our reality and never will be.

That calorie-counting machine is, in terms of calorie analysis, the most sophisticated operation I've ever witnessed but I could not help but ask the question: Does it work? Are you getting results? It felt awkward to ask (even for me, and I've spent my life being awkward). The answer was no; they had less than a 10 per cent success rate, for exactly the reason given above: because life happens. You have to understand that you are a human being, not a computer. It's not data in, data out. You're an animal;

you have emotions and you live with other people that have emotions and thoughts and different intentions and agendas, which means life can come at you and put any plan on the back-burner. Calorie counting has an almost heroic failure rate. So, rather than eating by numbers, go back to the basics and choose food that truly nourishes you, because not all calories are equal. You will not only feel amazing, but look amazing, too.

What does 'listening to my body' really mean?

A lot of people don't know they're sick because they've never been healthy. They are not in tune with their body at all. So many people think it is normal to wake up feeling tired, miserable, achy, bloated and gassy. It's not normal; it's just common. Normal is to wake up feeling energized, happy and recharged. Often people don't realize they have an issue with certain foods because they are just so numb from a general feeling of poor health and unhappiness.

This leads me to a story I often tell... An imaginary client wakes up every morning, has a quick bowl of cereal, gets dressed for work and walks to the bus stop, where she headbutts the wall 10 times, before searching through her bag for a headache tablet. It makes her feel a little better, but she is constantly on the search for a more effective headache tablet. What does this woman really need? A better headache tablet, or to change her behaviour and stop headbutting the wall?

Believe it or not, many of us are doing this in the way we think about what we eat — we have a behaviour that is causing an issue and so we search for a pill, a person, a book or a diet to change us. All we need to do is stop headbutting the wall. Anyone out there eating low-fat yoghurts, or doughnuts, or three gluten-free muffins a day, or pasta every night — you're headbutting the wall. Instead, follow this blueprint for health and choose foods that work for you.

I know it can be scary to realize that it's all in your own hands and that no one and nothing else can change this for you. It's all on you. Once you realize that, you can really change your life.

Next, you need to recognize how your body communicates with you. This includes gas (we're all friends here, so let's say 'farts'), tiredness, bad skin, moodiness, irritability, bloating, aches and pains, inflammation and mild depression.

If this is your 'normal', you need to change, because, if you don't, you'll only get more sick. Understand that these symptoms are your body's way of communicating with you.

Rhaya Jordan: Listening to your body can be scary or unfamiliar at first, but essentially, if you can tune in to your body and eat only when you are hungry and stop when you are full, your health and appearance will transform.

I work with obese clients and many of them eat in a trance. They eat until the food runs out, not until their body tells them to stop. To feel and look 'healthy', you need to flip that on its head. You need to stop when your body wants you to stop, not when the food runs out. It's not easy to do. One great way of starting this is to eat without your phone, laptop or any other distraction nearby. Your body whispers to you all the time, and if you are too busy or distracted, you won't hear it. So, when you eat, concentrate on just that. Be curious about what your body is saying to you. If you can do this, your body will help bring you back to balance faster than anything. Everything you need to be well and to achieve a healthy weight is there in your hard-wiring; you just need to pay attention.

It's important to learn the difference between listening to your body and giving in to cravings. Cravings will leave you feeling a bit jangly and desperate, and normally you can judge if it's a craving by the quality of the food that you are after. If you have a lot of cravings, make life easier and don't put yourself in harm's way. So, if you often crave chocolate, don't keep it in the house. Grease the track in the direction you want to go. When you feel satisfied and content after eating, that's when you've been listening to your body.

Look at what you eat and know that you will feel the effect within a few hours. If you eat a low-nutrient, high-sugar, highly processed meal, you will feel terrible within 30 minutes. As I've said before, you won't be able to recognize this if you are on a constant rollercoaster of eating toxic foods. So try the Bodyism Two-week Blueprint (see pages 88–91) as an introduction and then, when you add more foods back in, check in with how your body is communicating with you. If one or more of those negative symptoms are happening, think about what you have eaten and look at what it may be that is causing this reaction. Some of the common trigger foods are wheat, dairy, sugar and highly processed foods.

Why should I choose organic?

The fact that there is even a debate about whether or not organic is better is completely insane. So let's just keep it very simple: we know that pesticides are harmful to human beings, so you tell me which is better — a fruit that has pesticides on it, or a fruit that doesn't? We know without a doubt that the hormones used in non-organic meat are harmful to humans. So ask yourself this: which is better — meat with harmful hormones in it, or organic meat that doesn't have hormones in it? It really is that simple. It is more expensive to buy organic meat, so the way I deal with this is to have it less often. If you can't find organic, talk to the butcher and find out where their meat is sourced, or find a local farmers' market and do your research.

A study reported by Menus of Change stated that, 'In 1960, the total annual U.S. expenditures for food were estimated at $74 billion. This was roughly three times as much as the total expenditures that same year of $27 billion for healthcare. Fast-forward to 2013. U.S. citizens spent $1.42 trillion on food and $2.9 trillion on healthcare, flipping the ratio, with healthcare spending now twice that of food.' Invest in your health now and save on your healthcare bill later in life.

What makes a food 'healthy'?

An important factor in a food being healthy is your attitude towards it and how you are eating it. So, rather than thinking about what's healthy and what's not, start to think about being kind to yourself. With that attitude, you will naturally gravitate towards the food that works for you, energizes you and helps you achieve that 'perfect' body. 'What is the perfect body?' I hear you ask. There are people who are severely overweight or underweight and completely happy, but it is a medical reality that they are not healthy. There are others who have a wonderfully healthy body, but they are riddled with shame and guilt, so they are unhappy with it. Your body becomes perfect when it's healthy and happy.

What is a 'cheat meal'?

I used to swear by a cheat meal. My definition of a cheat meal is 'indulging in whatever you want'. (For me, that would be a chocolate and peanut-butter cake.) The science suggests that, if you eat a super-strict 'clean' diet all week long and then let off steam and indulge in one cheat meal, it ramps up your metabolism so you wake up leaner the next day. I'll admit, I was once a huge advocate of this and loved the whole idea of my cheat meal. The reality, however, was that it became a slight obsession for me. Halfway through the 'meal', I'd start to feel rubbish, my teeth would start to tingle and I'd feel uncomfortable in my skin. It wasn't pleasurable at all. But it was something that I had a psychological dependence on. I felt like it was part of my job to have my cheat meal.

The way that I nourish myself now is to ensure everything I eat is a joy. I'm not 'strict' any more because I really do live by the one rule of being kind to myself. I choose foods that nourish me,

make me feel good and are delicious and abundant. Living by that philosophy, I genuinely don't feel the psychological need for a cheat meal, and don't have to blow off steam, because I'm happy with how I'm eating, how I'm feeling and how I'm looking. How I eat during the week is not something I feel I have to 'endure' until I get to have the joy of my cheat meal. I feel balanced because there is so much more abundance in my diet. I have real carbs with my meals, like brown rice or beans — as I mentioned before, I used to think it was a 'treat' to do that. I had created a really joyless cycle and was living a 'when' life rather than a 'now' life. I used to think, 'I'll be happy when it's the weekend,' but now I think, 'I'm happy right now,' because food needs to be celebrated.

Now might be a good time to check some of your internal conversations. So, if there are thoughts in your head saying, 'I'll be happy when I lose weight,' or, 'I'll be happy when I get this job,' whatever it is, let that go and let yourself be happy now. Of course, sometimes life gets in the way, but, if you can, make a conscious choice to be happy right now.

If you choose to be kind to yourself right now, that horrible cycle of denial and indulgence will end. It is truly better to live without restriction and instead choose foods which make you feel good every day.

Are supplements a waste of money?

The short, truthful, correct answer is no — unless they are, in which case don't waste your money. What does that mean? In the world of supplements, there is no such thing as a bargain. If you're buying fish oils in a sale bin, then they are not going to work. That's the truth. If you're buying a protein powder in a four-kilo bucket with lightning bolts and a picture of some guy with veins popping out of his muscles and eyeballs, then it's probably going to be bad for you. Generally, cheap supplements, almost without exception, are a waste of money. In the supplement world, you really do get what you pay for.

Good-quality, ethically sourced, well-researched supplements do have an essential place in the

modern diet and here's why: food quality today isn't what it was 500 or even 100 years ago because of modern farming methods that have been in place since the end of the Second World War (it has got progressively worse since then). The fertilizers and pesticides we use force food to grow quicker, but with fewer nutrients. Soil quality has rapidly deteriorated and so have the nutrient levels in our food. I wish I could say you can get all of the nutrients you need from the food that you eat, but I'd be lying. It's not the truth, and anyone who says it is must be living in a commune in an organic field — in which case, all power to you. If you've got a job and you live with the stress of paying your rent or mortgage and all of the other stuff that most of us are privileged enough to live with, then let's get real. Every now and then, you just have to blend up a shake, drink it down and be grateful for it.

The reason people should take supplements is to boost or nourish their body in an achievable way, where it might otherwise be lacking, for whatever reason. Food quality isn't what it once was, and the sad reality is that we all need to supplement our diets. In fact, we need a new word for them, because the reality is that nowadays, supplements are essential. People need them.

As with everything, though, there is a balance. One of our trainers was once advised by a medical professional to take 'lots of vitamin D', so he started doing so and very soon began to feel really unwell. He had some tests and they showed that he had toxic levels of vitamin D in his system. He was taking so many different supplements that he messed up his digestive system, suffered from erectile dysfunction and lost his libido — all from doing too much of a 'good thing'. He had taken far too much. So, you've got to be mindful and aware of what you are taking as well as how much.

Rhaya Jordan: We burn through our nutrients faster when we are experiencing stress, modern pollution and lack of sleep. Supplements can bridge the gap in the modern world. A bad diet and supplements will not have a good outcome, but supplements can really turbo-charge a good diet.

Rhaya Jordan: It's a complete maze, so the simplest way to choose a supplement that is truly beneficial is to put a human you trust into the equation. Go to a health-food store and speak to someone who knows what they are doing. Look for some real food in the supplement's ingredient list (e.g. herbs, spices, berries etc.). The Bodyism supplements are the best I've ever seen.

What should I look for in a supplement?

There is so much dishonesty in the supplement industry, which is why, when I was creating the Bodyism supplements, I needed to make sure the products could be trusted. I continue to make sure that the supplements are made fairly and that the ingredients they claim to contain are actually contained. With products like these, you need to have someone who is accountable and putting their name to them. Our range of Bodyism supplements were each made with a specific result in mind: to improve sleep, help you go to the toilet, improve your skin or improve libido. Supplements create a simple, time-effective, achievable way of getting everything you need to nourish you. And making a shake with supplements is a symptom of the modern world — not everyone has the time to grow a cucumber and sing to it.

A word of warning: if you're taking a really good-quality protein supplement and a supergreen mix, but then you combine it with a banana, a mango and a pineapple, the sugar content of that smoothie is going to skyrocket. Be aware of what you are mixing your supplement with. Try almond milk or coconut milk, some greens (I'm talking spinach or cucumber, not broccoli), and be very aware of the amount of sugar you are putting in there. It comes back to balance. Fruit is great for you, but in excess it is high in sugar, so be mindful — you can't eat 30 bananas and expect to be nourished.

Which ingredients should you avoid in a supplement?

Look for fillers, which are all extremely difficult to absorb and basically just awful for you! These include hydrogenated oils, such as soybean oil, which is just a source of trans fats; they are very cheap and absolutely terrible for you. Also watch out for talc or magnesium silicate, and titanium dioxide.

Look for secret sugars: maltose, sucrose, fructose...

Check the type of protein. Vegan protein (rice, hemp and pea) is easiest to digest, so I always recommend that to my clients. Whey protein can work well, but it is made from cow's milk, so those with lactose intolerances may find it doesn't suit them.

See how you feel. As always, listen to your body. If the supplement makes you feel energized and recharged then keep on with it! If you feel bloated, change the portion size or try another supplement.

Any ingredients you don't know, look them up.

What should I do if I'm craving sugar?

Have a glass of water! I know I sound like a party pooper, but I'm not kidding, because sometimes we crave sugar when we are really thirsty. It might also be your body saying you need more protein, carbs or fats in your meals — if you are under-eating or not choosing nourishing foods, I guarantee you will be craving a sweet fix. So, if you can bear it, rather than reaching for a cheap sugar hit, have some nuts instead or some cold meat or even a protein shake (but choose it wisely), or if you really want something sweet, go for fruit or dark/bittersweet chocolate. If you can nourish yourself with some form of protein, you will feel so much better than if you abuse your body with a highly processed, high-sugar snack.

What five 'healthy' foods am I eating that could be making me sick?

1. Raw vegan energy balls. Check the sugar content because, however they are dressed up, you could be consuming a huge amount of sugar without even realizing it. Try to find something genuinely healthy and nourishing, because these balls can send you on a sugar-craving rollercoaster (and result in a big sugar tantrum).

2. Smoothies from the supermarket. These can contain more sugar than a fizzy drink.

3. Green juices. Just because it's 'green' doesn't mean it's vegetable-rich and freshly pressed. Just like some smoothies, some of these 'green' juices contain about six apples with one spinach leaf. An apple is good for you, but not a whole tree in one go. Check the ingredients carefully.

4. Low-fat yoghurt. It tends to have loads of flavourings, thickeners and a lot of sugar. Go for full-fat, natural yoghurt and a packet of blueberries instead of a fruit yoghurt. Once again, please remember full-fat won't make you fat — it's more satisfying and will actually help curb your appetite.

5. Gluten-free food. Some of the 'free from' ranges out there are just processed, refined, super-expensive junk food. A slap in the face is gluten-free — it doesn't mean it's good for you. When someone holds up a gluten-free muffin as something healthy, my heart sinks. Often they've replaced the gluten with gums and upped the sugar content, neither of which is good for you.

What five things should I never eat after a workout?

1. A gluten-free muffin. No matter what it says, whether it's got refined sugar or 'pretend' sugar, it's going to stop that fat-burning process within your body immediately. When you do cardio, you will burn fat afterwards until the very second that sugar hits your mouth, because your insulin spikes immediately and that stops you burning fat. If you do a resistance circuit, you will burn fat for up to three hours after you finish working out — or until the very second that sugar goes into your system. Instead, reach for a protein shake which doesn't have a load of sugar in it.

2. Energy drinks. Especially the fluorescent ones (in case you didn't realize it already, you should never drink anything fluorescent) — they are a chemical cocktail of toxic rubbish. These toxic drinks spike your insulin levels, giving you a short-term sugar rush, which then puts you on that unhealthy rollercoaster of feeling 'tired and wired' and will, almost without exception, create cravings and poor food choices for the rest of the day. Not to mention all the other funky stuff it does to your body.

3. Fruit smoothies. If your 'why' for working out is to feel healthy and lose weight (which is absolutely fine), don't sabotage your best intentions and undo all of the effort that you've just made by consuming a load of sugar dressed up in a fruit smoothie. If it's crammed with pineapple or apple juice, it's not a healthy smoothie and it's not a healthy 'green' juice either. Shop-bought smoothies dress up as your 'friends', but actually they're the 'mean girls' who just want you to put on weight.

4. Chocolate cake. It may surprise you, but chocolate cake is one of the most popular snacks people buy at their health club. In a study published in the May 2014 issue of Marketing Letters, people who were told a 2-km walk was 'exercise' ate 35 per cent more chocolate pudding afterwards than those who thought the same stroll was a 'scenic walk'. The mentality is 'I've just worked out, so now I'm going to reward myself with this chocolate cake.' Now you've learnt the science around sugar post-exercise (see point 1), you'll know better. You can't out-exercise an unhealthy diet; it just doesn't work like that. Also, think about why you are reaching for the chocolate cake — if it's because you see chocolate as a reward and exercise as a punishment, then you need to make an effort to change the story and find exercise that you actually enjoy.

5. Energy bars. Most of them are packed with natural sugars in the form of dates, which have an incredibly high GI load that not only stops the fat-burning process immediately, but will also contribute to weight gain. Professional athletes may require these short fixes from time to time, but, unless you are also in training, it doesn't apply to you.

How do I know when I've eaten too much?

This is where tuning in to your body becomes so powerful. Rather than associating food with a fearful mind, learn to eat with a calm, relaxed mind. When I was dealing with my obsessive behaviour surrounding food, I had a mantra that I would say in my head before I ate: 'I am safe. I am loved. I am in perfect health. I live in abundance.' (This is fine to say in your head, but don't say it out loud because apparently it 'disturbs the other customers!') Saying those affirmations helped me remember to be mindful every time I ate.

Just taking 30 seconds to tune in to how you are feeling before you eat and halfway through your meal can stop you from overeating. The easiest way to stop eating when you're satisfied, rather than over full, is to chew your food thoroughly. I notice customers eating at the café and it's striking to see the differences in how they do it. Some people eat so fast, with their phone in their hand, and it's a vacant, mindless experience. Sometimes, I'll sit next to them (not in a creepy way) and ask, 'How's the food?' What's surprising is that so many haven't even thought about it. If this sounds like you, then work at it; it has the power to change your entire wellbeing.

⫴MOVEMENT

'Movement is magical.'

Don't be one of those annoying people that says, 'I just hate exercise.' You don't, it's just you need to find what exercise you really enjoy. I've lost count of the number of people I've turned from hating exercise to valuing their body, cherishing moving it and feeling incredible.

I've included some Bodyism circuits in this chapter. You will see in the Bodyism Two-week Blueprint (see pages 88–91) how to create a full workout using these circuits. Always remember to start with Prehab Circuit (see pages 62–63) and end with the Regenerate Circuit (see pages 72–73). Normally, I would add two of the other circuits, repeated two to three times.

Why is movement a pillar of health?

Movement is medicine, not just for the body, but for the mind, too. Our bodies were made to move, so we deserve to do that. Almost every day, a new study is published proving the benefits of exercise. The benefits aren't just physical, but psychological, too. In April 2014, the University of Eastern Finland found that physical activity can protect against dementia in old age. The researchers found that participants who engaged in physical activity at least twice a week had a much lower risk of dementia than those who were less active.

Movement is directly related to cognitive ability (yes, it will literally make you smarter), a decreased risk of mental illness and degenerative diseases, and generally leads to you being happier and healthier for longer. If you need any more convincing of why movement is a pillar of health, then this book isn't for you. Put it down and swap it for a doughnut.

When I say 'movement', I mean exercise. That doesn't mean lifting weights until your ears bleed or putting on hot pants and jumping up and down for an hour and a half every day. It can be a walk with a really intelligent, gentle stretching programme and a couple of body-weight resistance circuits per week — that's all you need for a long, healthy, happy life. Imagine if every day you went for a 45-minute walk, did some gentle stretching and a few squats and lunges alongside eating and sleeping well — you'd be well on the road to being healthy, slim and full of energy. That person could be you. You don't even have to do anything crazy to get there; you just have to be kind to your body.

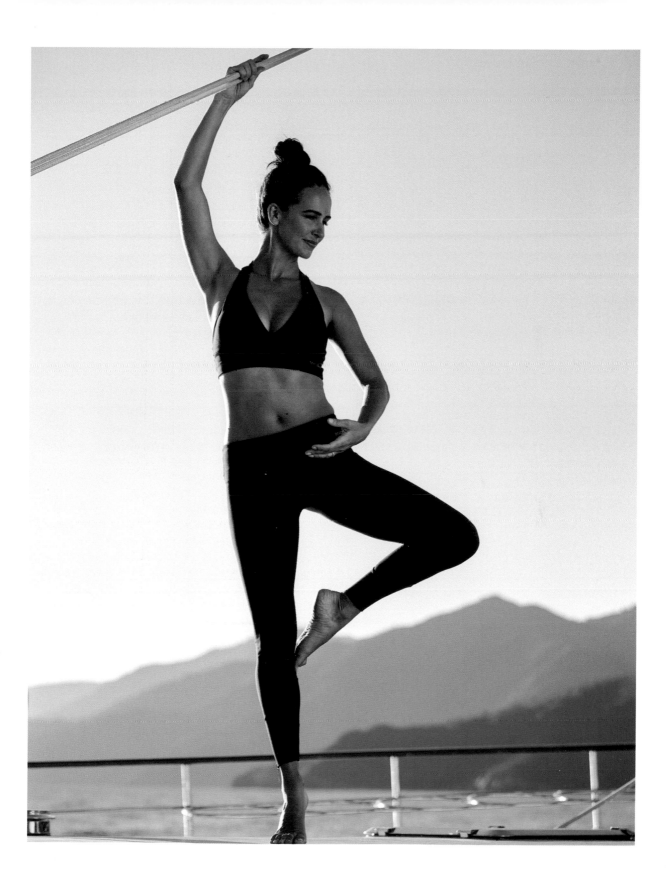

How often should I move?

This is the question that I always get asked. Perhaps a better question is, 'How often do I have the privilege and the joy of moving?' The answer is that your body loves to move, so be grateful you can move your body and do it every day.

Find time to move every day in different ways. Don't just stick to the gym — carry your children, walk in the park or offer to give someone a piggyback to work from the bus stop (only kidding... maybe don't do that). You get the point. Embrace change. I am a creature of habit and I'm really comfortable being comfortable. But, when I've opened my mind and tried something new, I've never regretted it (apart from that one time I decided to join the new tap-dancing club... I really regret that).

If we think of exercise in the same way that we think about food, it will illustrate why balance and variety is so important. Is broccoli good for us? Yes, absolutely it is. So, should we just eat broccoli every day and nothing else? Absolutely not. That would be really stupid and unhealthy. If you did that, you would have an eating disorder.

So, we ask the same question with exercise: is running good for you? Yes, it is. Is it all I should ever do? Absolutely not. Just like nutrition — be balanced about it.

I am soon to be 42 and I've never been in better shape. I probably train less than ever, but I mix things up. I lift weights for 20 minutes twice a week, I do yoga and my great joy and hobby is jiu-jitsu, which I do three times a week.

We've included circuits in this book, which will show you some really safe, effective exercises that will get you started. Sign up to something new, be careful and constantly come back to the question, 'Am I being kind to myself?'

Why do I need to warm up?

What we consider 'warming up' is not what it was 10 years ago: it doesn't simply mean 20 minutes on the treadmill; it means intelligent, targeted movement prep.

It's called 'movement prep' because it literally prepares your body for movement. It's dedicated to getting the right muscles 'switched on' so that you achieve results in less time, prevent injury and optimize your workout.

So, hip extensions switch on your glutes (and help perk your butt), plank variations switch your abdominals on, supermans switch on your postural muscles and connect your arms and legs with your abdominals. All of these movements have a really powerful reason behind them and they are a simple, effective way of preparing your body for whatever movement you are about to do.

Movement prep amplifies your workout and obviously makes it much safer. You need to get your body and mind ready to move if you want to enhance your performance and prevent injury.

How long should I train for?

I have had requests from people who want to train for 90 minutes or two hours. The fact is, if you're training for that long, you are doing it wrong. You are not doing it smart enough. You can make significant progress with your body, without damaging it, by simply working the three aspects of movement intelligently:

1. Balance. Movements that challenge your balance include single leg work, single arm work, certain yoga poses and even closing your eyes while doing a familiar movement, like a squat or a lunge, or even a push-up. You'll be surprised how much more demanding that is.

2. **Strength.** This can be anything from lifting weights to bodyweight exercises, such as squats, single lunges, press-ups, or, if you're ready for it, handstands.

3. **Cardio.** This includes the full spectrum, from sustained cardio, such as a long walk in the park, to high-intensity cardio, such as sprints in the gym.

A really good, balanced programme will incorporate all three of these. Even if you are training for a marathon, it is important to implement all three aspects of exercise. If you just run without doing joint stabilization, strength work and skill-based balance work, there is a greater chance of injury through faulty movement patterns and unstable joints.

Just remember, as we've said many times before, life is long (hopefully), so a workout should amplify your enjoyment of it, rather than break your body down or become joyless and obsessive. Nourish your body.

Is running good or bad?

It's both. It's great because it's free, you can start immediately and you can do it just about anywhere in the world. On the flip side, it often becomes obsessive, destructive and can cause long-term damage if you overdo it. It's one of the first things Hollywood stylists and anti-ageing experts will tell you to stop doing, because of the effect it has on your face (it causes sagging) and the amount of oxidative stress it puts on your system. So running is great if it's your only option, but there are so many better ways of getting a healthy, happy body. If you really do love running, then go for it, enjoy it, but please be balanced and include some strength training in your workout (if you're running in the park, just find a bench and do some triceps dips, lunges and squats). And always do your movement prep.

Is cycling good or bad?

Cycling is a repetitive movement pattern, so it can reduce your athletic ability in terms of motor skills and coordination. Cyclists as well as rowers have been known to suffer from a significant amount of back pain. I'm saying this so you are aware of the side effects, as well as the positives. What I'm not saying is, 'Avoid cycling.' It's fantastic, as long as it's part of a balanced, intelligent programme that nourishes and works your entire body. If this is your chosen sport and hobby, and it brings you great joy, then brilliant, but incorporate movement prep and make sure you add the Bodyism circuits into your week.

How long will it take me to see results?

It depends what you mean by 'results'. As we know, any change that happens in your body, happens in your mind first. So, the second you commit to being kind to yourself and living a long, happy, healthy life is the very moment that you get the most important and powerful transformation: the change in your mind. The rest is easy and you will then start to see the results in your body very quickly. The changes that you see in your body are just a side effect of the wonderful changes that you make in your mind, and when you truly begin to enjoy the process and appreciate that life is a beautiful journey, as opposed to a series of destinations, not only do you stop thinking about results in terms of body-fat percentage or a number on a scale, but your body transforms at a breathtaking rate; this is when the fastest and most dramatic changes happen. The tricky thing about this is that you only see it when you stop looking for it.

In order to achieve life-changing results in an intelligent way, focus on the four pillars of health. So many people just focus on one pillar of health. For example, they might exercise to an extreme level, but then they aren't sleeping, their mindset is all wrong and they're eating badly. It's not the fastest or most intelligent way of doing it. Instead, when you begin to calmly see what needs to be done in all four pillars of health (and, by the way, this doesn't take long to do) and you work on them equally and intelligently, your body will transform so much faster. The desperately miserable person on the spinning bike or in the middle of a hard-core exercise class is doing long-term damage, working harder and taking longer than the Bodyism champion. You now know that you don't need to go all-out on a spinning bike to look and feel great — just try not to be smug about it.

Why is rest important?

I always thought resting was me being lazy, but rest is when the magic happens. Those rest days are when your body recharges, regenerates and actually when it really burns fat and creates long, lean muscle — it's when everything is optimized.

Rest days can take many different forms. So, if three or four times a week you are training to a more intense level, on the other days, just go for a nice walk, or do some gentle yoga, or, if you can, book yourself in for a massage. The amount of rest you take depends on the level of exercise you are doing. So, for me, I do jiu-jitsu three times a week, which is fairly high intensity, and on the other days I walk or do yoga or play with the kids. Sunday is my day of complete rest from any kind of organized exercise — it's also when I try and have either a warm bath or a massage (if I'm really lucky).

How do I know if I'm overtraining?

As I've said, movement is medicine. So, just like all medicine, you can overdose on it. Exercise is wonderful for you, but when you do too much of it, you can ruin your body. It can cause injury, create hormonal imbalances and lower your immune system. So what are the signs that you are overtraining?

1. Exhaustion. In simple terms, if you have a constant feeling of exhaustion, that is not a good thing. It's great to really push yourself every now and then, and feeling exhausted from your workout can be a really fulfilling experience. It becomes a problem when it is happening four times a week and you walk out of the gym completely depleted, especially when you combine this with poor food choices. You are depleting your system and undernourishing yourself, and eventually you will get sick and injured. This isn't an 'if', it's a 'when'. It happens all the time: people burn out. It's great to train and move and really test your limits, but do it intelligently and make sure you nourish your body with good-quality food and good-quality rest.

2. Poor food choices. People who overtrain tend to make poor food choices alongside their workouts. Either they 'reward' themselves with processed foods or a sugar-filled 'treat' that has no protein or nutritional value — and then push themselves to work even harder in the gym the next day — or they choose foods that won't allow their body to recover and replenish. So it might be they'll have a coffee and some steamed lettuce leaves (thinking that's the only way to lose weight) and their body will go into starvation insurance straight away. They might get short-term results for a little while, but it won't ever work for the long term.

3. Niggling Injuries. Another sign you are overtraining is constant niggling injuries. This is your body's very powerful way of telling you what you are doing is not working. Don't ignore it; listen to it. That constant pain in your knee, hip, back or wherever is your body telling you something needs to be looked at, so if you are training through that and you don't make your living from doing exercise as a professional athlete, there is a real issue there. Pain is another way of your body communicating with you. So take a rest for a second and find someone that can help you with that injury. Lower back pain can come from not enough exercise because your muscles are weak, or it can come from too much exercise

because you are doing the wrong thing constantly. So if you are exercising frequently but notice aches and pains, please do not ignore it. This happens a lot to keen spinners because often people compromise their posture on the spinning bike which can put unnecessary pressure on your back.

4. Dreading training. If you're dreading it and there's no fun anymore, something is not working for you. You need to keep searching for what you love.

5. Prioritizing exercise above everything, always. Let exercise be a part of your life; don't let it get in the way of your life. There are people who will choose to exercise over anything and everything. Don't miss out on the other things happening in your life in order to do an extra session at the gym, because you'll regret it later. Make sure you are choosing exercise because you actually want to do it and it feels right. I remember being in a meeting in New York and I was chatting to an agent there. He told me he was going spinning in the morning and in the evening. He was proudly addicted. Without a doubt, that kind of punishing schedule of hard core, high-intensity exercise does long-term damage. Remember, your body loves to move every day, but that doesn't mean you have to go to a high-intensity class — walking is just as amazing.

6. Weight gain. The biology of overtraining often creates a high production of cortisol (the stress hormone shown to dump fat on the front of the tummy). You can literally run yourself fat. Sometimes, I work with clients who are not eating enough and are exercising too much, which prevents them from losing weight, as they are in a constant state of starvation insurance. Their bodies are not willing to let go of fat. That's where the magic of being intelligent about the four pillars really comes into play. If you nourish yourself properly by eating more good-quality foods, your body will feel amazing and will not be in a constant state of fight or flight. When you go to these crazy high-intensity classes, you are working against your body, not with it.

Top Tip Manage your movement habit. Many people are addicted to exercise. They are ruining their bodies because of it. Whatever belief is driving you to do that amount of exercise needs to be addressed: it's about managing that situation and always coming back to being kind to yourself. I'm addicted to exercise, but as with any recovering addict, I manage it. If, like me, you don't feel good if you haven't exercised, it doesn't mean that you then have to do spinning or High-intensity Interval Training every day. Change your mindset and remind yourself that any movement is great — a long walk, a swim, yoga, a dance class, boxing, lifting — and will keep you feeling brilliant. Make sure it's balanced. I've been stuck in a rut of doing the same thing every day. It's all about scheduling, so put in your diary: today is yoga, tomorrow is weights etc. Once it's written down, have a look at it. If it's all high intensity, change it up.

If you're an exercise addict, you'll understand completely what I'm saying here. If you're not and this makes no sense to you at all, then don't worry, move along because this doesn't apply to you. Make the changes that will help you and be guided by the principles of being kind to yourself.

PS: If it's Friday and you haven't moved since last Thursday's exercise class and you're wondering if you are overdoing it, you're not. This word of warning is not for you.

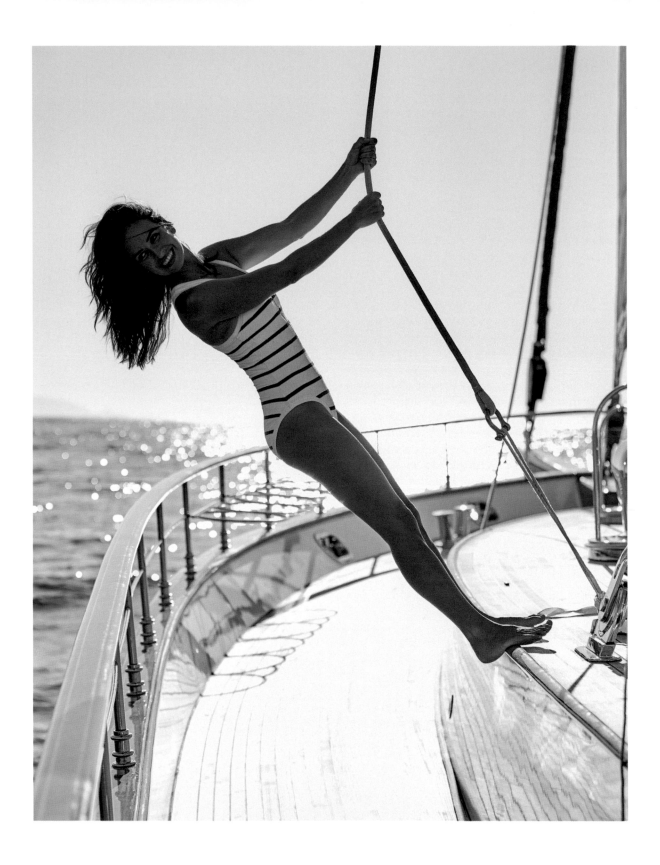

How do you get back on track after a big slip?

Living well needs to become part of your life, rather than controlling your life. You don't need to spend hours making healthy food; you don't need to train for an hour a day. You just need to move your body every day (our circuits will take you less than 20 minutes) and eat nourishing foods.

When Chrissy had our daughter, Charlotte, the first thing she did was walk. She didn't need to start with yoga or pilates — just walking and getting in touch with her body was exactly what she needed.

Christiane Duigan: My biggest tip is to start slowly. When I began exercising again, I started off doing one or two hip extensions at a time, then I slowly built it up. Alongside this, I walked every day and did pelvic floor exercises. I kept an eye on my posture, because good posture makes you look slimmer and strengthens your core, which helps your stomach muscles fuse back together. I didn't need to lift weights because I was lifting Charlotte all the time. I didn't deprive myself, I just ate healthy foods (I didn't cut out any food groups), and I listened to my body. I took my time and I'm glad I did, because when weight comes off slowly and steadily, it stays off for longer. Remember, you don't need to rush. Be kind and respectful to yourself.

Will exercise ever feel fun?

It's all about how you approach something. When you realize that you are lucky to be able to move, it changes things. Remember, exercise doesn't mean you have to wear hot pants and dance around like a maniac for an hour. It can take the form of a long walk, squats, lunges, press-ups and dips in your living room, or going to your local gym and connecting with other human beings. When it's not fun, change it up.

For me, surfing and jiu-jitsu are constantly inspiring, creative and fun. Of course, there are times when they're challenging, but I value those times too, because I can transcend any difficulties and then transfer that determination into my life. It creates strength and the ability to keep going when I'm uncomfortable or feel like giving up. I've learnt so much from being a very bad surfer, trying to get out through big waves and never giving up. Every time I do that, it makes me stronger and more determined. It's the same with jiu-jitsu: I don't have a natural talent, but what I've developed is a real strength of purpose and will. I won't give up; sometimes I lose (in fact, often I lose), but I never get beaten (what this means is I won't quit), and that inspires me in my daily life. Find the value in exercising and moving.

Why do I lose weight on holiday?

Because you're relaxed. This is the shortest, most correct, most complete answer. The science remains the same: when your body and mind let go (and stop stressing and obsessing), it not only enables you to lose weight, but also ongoing intolerances can just disappear. It is a really incredible example of how what you think can totally affect how you feel and how you look. Try to take what you notice about your behaviour on holiday/vacation back home with you. For example, on holiday/vacation, we always spend so much more time enjoying our meals. We eat slowly and calmly, which gives us our best chance to really listen to our bodies. A holiday/vacation takes us away from our daily stresses, enabling us to metabolize better, digest better and be more mindful than normal.

How do you know when to go from losing weight to maintaining a healthy weight?

What's amazing about the human body is you don't need to worry about that. When you're nourishing yourself, moving intelligently and being kind to yourself, your body will go to its ideal weight. As soon as you are treating it right, you won't need to restrain yourself; your body will just know and you'll feel energized and 'right'. If you are being kind to yourself, you will be listening to what your body wants and not feel like you are restricting yourself in any way. The moment you are in tune with your body, you will not need to think about losing weight.

Where do I start if I'm severely overweight, have joint problems and lost any motivation?

Firstly, you are not alone. So many people are in exactly the same situation, or very similar. By following the Blueprint, so many issues you are dealing with will disappear and it will happen much quicker than you can imagine. By nourishing your body, by doing some gentle movement every single day, you will start to notice profound changes, not just in how you look, but also how you feel.

'Be more powerful than all of your excuses.'

How can I lift my butt?

Resistance bands are one of the only pieces of equipment we use. They are incredibly effective and are such an intelligent way to lift your butt (exercises can include band-walking and hip extensions) without overworking the quads (which is a very common problem for many people who sit at a desk every day). The other great thing about the bands is they enable you to work your butt without damaging your knees, hips or ankles. It actually helps stabilize those joints, too. We've got elite athletes who warm up with these bands. If you don't have the bands (or can't get them because they haven't invented the Internet where you live), then hip extensions and squat thrusts are your butt's best friend. Another great thing to do when you're on the go is to actively squeeze your glutes whenever you can. If you're ever standing in line at the supermarket, waiting to pick up your kids from school or are at the bus stop, just squeeze your butt for 10 seconds as hard as you can and then rest for 10 seconds. Honestly, if you do this every day, it will help you get a smoking hot butt. (Don't do this while you walk, because it will look like you are urgently looking for a toilet...)

How do I get a flat tummy?

A flat tummy won't make you happy, but being happy will give you a flat tummy.

I trained a client who would always say, 'I'm training until I get there.' I would ask her, 'Until you get where?' and she'd say, 'Until I lose weight and get abs.' I said to her, 'You'll never get there because you are always *here*.'

Please remember, you are always where you are in the present moment; it's not *when*, it's only *now* and *here*. My client was smart and very quickly became less obsessed and realized that *when* doesn't exist.

All the things that make people happy — less stress, nourishing foods, a good night's sleep — will lead to a flat tummy as a by-product. Also, a flat tummy is way more than doing ab crunches. In fact, your stomach is almost like a second brain. It is no accident that they call it 'gut instinct' or a 'gut feeling'. So much of it is emotionally driven. So, if you can find ways to relieve your stress, you'll see the effects in your tummy. Also, if you can heal your gut, it solves so many seemingly unrelated problems — emotionally, physically and hormonally. If you can get your digestion right, everything else is easy (see the Nutrition chapter, pages 24–45).

How can I make my legs long and lean?

Can you give the appearance of longer, leaner legs? Absolutely.

If the majority of your exercise is spinning, squats and lunges, running and other shortening exercises, chances are your legs won't look long and lean. To achieve that long, lean aesthetic, you need to add lengthening exercises, such as yoga, pilates and ballet, as well as postural exercises (the quickest way of giving the appearance of weight loss), with just a small amount of cardio and lifting. Cardio includes long, sustained movement, like walking and also quick high-intensity cardio bursts which raise your heart rate. Your attitude to exercise will be reflected in your body; so if you're obsessive and only lifting weights, your body will reflect that.

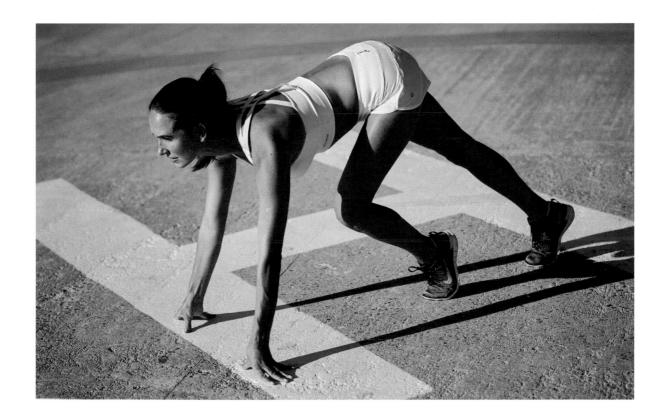

Will weightlifting make women bulky?

The science would suggest not. It can't make women bulky because of their relatively low levels of testosterone and the way they are built, biochemically and mechanically. But you have to be intelligent about it. If you don't want to look like a bodybuilder, don't train like a bodybuilder. If you're doing heavy-weighted squats, deadlifts and lunges every day, eventually your legs will adapt. The problem is most women are quad-dominant (they activate their quads more than their glutes and their hamstrings) because we all spend so much time sitting down. Big quads give the appearance of bulky legs much more than anything else. So, if you incorporate lengthening exercises like yoga, Pilates and stretching into weight sessions, and add some quick cardio bursts, that's how you get results which will reduce the likelihood of bulking up. That's not to say that lifting weights will definitely bulk you up, but you need to learn to manage your programme well. If you lift two to three times a week, it will keep your bones strong and healthy, help you maintain lean muscle mass and keep your connective tissue strong. If you're lifting to the point of injury and exhaustion, pull it back. You are your own expert.

Final word on movement

Please do not underestimate the importance of stretching. Give your body time to come back to its normal rhythm after exercising, so you can feel refreshed, mindful and re-energized when you finish your workout (our Regenerate Circuit on pages 72–73 will do just that).

BODYISM EXERCISES

Here are some of our best-loved exercise circuits. As I always say, you are your own expert so choose the exercises that you enjoy the most, mix and match, and find the joy in moving your body. Always remember to start with the Prehab Circuit (pages 62–63) to warm up those muscles and end with the Regenerate Circuit (pages 72–73) to, well, regenerate.

Each time you exercise, choose two of the circuits from the selection in the following pages (Perky Butt, Long Lean Legs, Flat-Tummy or Perfect Posture) and repeat the first circuit twice. Next, complete the Quick Cardio Burst (opposite). Now, for the second circuit — do it twice — then follow immediately with a second round of the Quick Cardio Burst. Finish with the Regenerate Circuit and always remember, your body loves to move.

Follow the at-a-glance chart below once you are in the swing of things.

WARM UP

**1x Prehab Circuit
(page 62–63)**

CIRCUITS

**2x circuit of your choice
(pages 64–71)**

**1x Quick Cardio Burst
(opposite)**

**2x circuit of your choice
(pages 64–71)**

**1x Quick Cardio Burst
(opposite)**

COOL DOWN

**1x Regenerate Circuit
(pages 72–73)**

QUICK CARDIO BURST

Hand Walkouts
(30 seconds)

1. Stand up straight with hands in the air.

2. Bring your hands down to the ground and walk them forward, until you are in a plank position. Make sure you brace your glutes and abs and then walk your hands further forward.

3. Reverse the movement by walking your hands back to the starting position and stand with your hands in the air again. Keep your head neutral with your spine.

4. Repeat, as fast as you can, for 30 seconds.

Mountain Climbers
(30 seconds)

1. Begin in a press-up position, with hands under shoulders, back flat, feet together and belly button drawn in.

2. Keep your core tight, bring one knee forward, towards your chest, then straighten your leg back out behind you.

3. Repeat with the opposite leg and continue for 30 seconds, as fast as you can.

Burpees, no jump
(30 seconds)

1. Stand up straight with your feet shoulder-width apart. Sink back into a squat position, with your backside pushed out, as if to sit down. Sink further, to go from a squat to a crouch.

2. Put your hands on the floor in front of you, shoulder-width apart.

3. Hop back with your feet, into a plank position. Make your body a straight line from your head to your ankles. Line up your shoulders with your wrists. Keep your body straight — don't arch your backside up or droop at the waist.

4. Bring your feet back to your hands with a quick hop.

5. Stand up to return to the starting position. Repeat, as fast as you can, for 30 seconds.

Alternating Disco Lunge
(30 seconds)

1. Begin standing in an upright position, with feet together and perfect posture (stand up straight, keep your back straight, with your ears over your shoulders and your shoulders over your hips. Look straight ahead and think tall, right through your spine and through the top of your head). Begin with your arms by your sides, with hands clenched, thumbs up.

2. Set your core by drawing in your belly button and step forward into a lunge.

3. As you lunge forward with your left foot, extend both arms above your head to make a Y shape. Land heel then toe and let your front knee bend forward.

4. Push back to the starting position with your arms by your sides. Repeat for 30 seconds.

Top Tip Repeat each exercise for 30 seconds and then rest for 15 seconds. Repeat the whole circuit four times. It's an awesome cardio burst.

PREHAB CIRCUIT

Hip Extension
(10–12 repetitions)

1. Lie on your back with your knees bent.

2. Exhale and roll your pelvis to lift your glutes and lower back off the ground. Try to create a straight line from your shoulders to your knees.

3. Pause at the top while squeezing your glutes, then reverse the movement, rolling each vertebra of the spine back to the starting position. Remember to use your glutes in this movement rather than over-working your lower back. Repeat 10–12 times.

Supermans
(10–12 repetitions, both sides)

1. Begin on your hands and knees with toes firmly pointed into the floor. Ensure your spine and neck are in a neutral position, with hands under shoulders and knees under hips.

2. Extend your right arm out in front of you alongside your head, thumb up, while you extend your left leg backwards toes still pointing down (imagine you are being pulled from either end).

3. Bring your arm and leg in underneath your torso simultaneously so they touch. Repeat 10–12 times before switching sides.

Top Tip Every time you do one of these circuits, make sure you hold your stomach in and really activate your glutes (clench your butt)!

Hip to Hamstring
(10 repetitions, both sides)

1. Place your left foot flat on the ground and your right knee on a soft pad or mat (on the ground).

2. Rest your left hand on the knee of your front leg.

3. Lean slightly forward with your torso, tighten your stomach, and contract the glute of your back leg.

4. Maintaining this position, shift your entire body slightly forward. Then move your hips backwards, straightening your front leg and moving forward with your torso to stretch the hamstring. Repeat 10 times before switching sides.

Thoracic Rotation with Adductor Stretch
(10 repetitions, both sides)

1. Start on all fours with your hands under your shoulders, one knee under your hip, the other straight out to the side with the foot against the floor.

2. With the hand on the same side as the outstretched leg, salute to your head, and rotate your torso through your shoulder blades so the elbow of your saluting arm points towards the ceiling (or sky).

3. Return back slowly, touch elbow to elbow, then return to the start position. Repeat 10 times before switching sides.

**Goddess to Relieve Squat
(12–15 repetitions)**

1. Stand with your arms straight out in front at shoulder height, feet wider than shoulder-width apart and toes pointed out at 45 degrees. Keep your core engaged by drawing your belly button in towards your spine.

2. Initiate the movement by pushing the hips back and bending the knees so you squat back and down until your thighs are parallel to the floor. Return to the standing position by pushing through the hips and the heels while keeping your torso upright. Repeat 12–15 times.

**Rainbow Slide with Gliders
(12–15 repetitions, both sides)**

1. Stand with your arms out in front of you, feet shoulder-width apart with your toes on a Bodyism gliding disc on each side. (If you don't have the discs, you could try using a small paper plate — it works in a similar way!)

2. Slide your left foot in front of you and then arc it out to the left, holding on to the disc as you go. Keep your right knee bent throughout.

3. Reverse the movement, returning briefly to the starting position whilst keeping your right knee bent. Repeat the sequence 12–15 times before repeating on the other foot.

Pike Adductor
(12–15 repetitions)

1. Step onto two Bodyism gliding discs (or small paper plates) and start in a pike position. With arms and legs straight, plant your hands directly under your shoulders to make your butt the highest point. Keep the weight in your hands and toes and relax your shoulders.

2. Tighten your core and glutes and drive your legs to a wide stance, taking the discs with you as you go. Reverse the movement back to the starting position. Repeat 12–15 times.

Hip Extension on Toes
(15 repetitions)

1. Lie on your back with both knees bent, toes on the ground and heels in the air.

2. Lift your hips off the ground, raising them as high as you can go, squeezing your glutes together and keeping your core tight.

3. Pause at the top for 1 second, then return to the start position. Repeat 15 times.

PERKY BUTT CIRCUIT

Tube Walking
(3 repetitions)

1. Stand in a quarter-squat position, with your feet hip-width apart and place a Bodyism mini band around your feet making sure it is taut (if you don't have a Bodyism band, you can use another exercise band).

2. Walk to the side with small steps for 10 strides and then walk back, leading with the opposite leg. Repeat this three times.

Rocket Lunge
(10 repetitions, both sides)

1. Take a step back with your left foot, bending both knees at 90 degrees, so your back knee hovers off the floor.

2. Extend both knees and transfer your weight on to your right foot. At the same time, lift up your left foot, bringing your knee to your chest while raising your arms to the ceiling.

3. Release your left leg from your chest and place it back on the floor in the starting lunge position. Repeat 10 times on each side.

Drop Step Lunge with Reach
(10 repetitions, both sides)

1. From a standing position with hands on hips, take a big step back with your right foot and move it behind the left foot. Once your right foot makes contact with the ground, square your hips, chest and feet so they are all facing forward.

2. Sit back slowly and drop your back knee towards the ground while reaching across your torso with your right hand. Feel the stretch in the outside of your thigh and your glutes. Keep your chest up and body squared, facing forward, the entire time.

3. Stand back up to return to the starting position. Repeat 10 times, then reset on the opposite side.

Sunrise Split Squat
(10 repetitions, both sides)

1. Stand in a staggered stance, with right foot in front of left, with your hands on your head.

2. Begin by lowering yourself down (not forward) until your left knee is almost touching the ground. Pause, then push yourself back up to starting position. Repeat 10 times with your right foot forward and then repeat with the left foot forward.

FLAT-TUMMY CIRCUIT

**Lunge Twist
(10 repetitions, both sides)**

1. Lunge forward; keep your hips facing forward, with your head still, arms out to the side parallel with the ground.

2. As you move down into the lunge, slowly rotate your torso over the lead leg, with your hands still out to the side. Keep your body upright, with your chest out and shoulders rolled back.

3. Rotate back to the middle and then return to the starting position. Repeat 10 times, then continue with the other leg.

**High Plank to Shin Tap
(10 repetitions, both sides)**

1. Start in high-plank position (just like traditional plank but with straight arms instead of them being bent at the forearm).

2. Lift your right hand off the floor and reach under your torso towards your left ankle (gently tapping the front of your foot or ankle, if possible).

3. Return the right hand to the floor and repeat with the opposite arm. Repeat 10 times on each side.

**Side Plank — Knee to Elbow
(10 repetitions, both sides)**

1. Come into a forearm side plank on your left side, with your left elbow resting on the floor below your shoulder.

2. Place your right arm behind your head and lift your right knee up towards your bent arm. Don't let your hips drop. Repeat 10 times on each side.

**The Body Saw with Gliding Discs
(10 repetitions)**

1. Start on the floor and come into a forearm plank, with your fists clenched or your palms facing up.

2. Place each foot on a Bodyism gliding disc. (If you don't have the discs, you could try using a small paper plate — it works in a similar way!)

3. Keeping your body in a straight line, press your forearms into the floor (forearms should not move) to push your body backwards, so your arms form a 60-degree angle.

4. Reverse the motion by pressing into your forearms to pull your body forwards, back to the start position. Repeat this 10 times.

Floor Slide
(10 repetitions)

1. Lie on your back with your legs flat and heels on the ground. (If you find this exercise difficult, begin with your knees bent and feet on the ground.)

2. Place both arms out at shoulder height on the floor, with elbows bent at 90 degrees.

3. Tuck in your chin, engage your torso and slowly slide both arms up along the floor towards your head, without letting your lower back, rib cage, shoulders or chin lift.

4. Stop at the top and slide your arms back to the starting position. Repeat 10 times.

Disco Lunge
(10 repetitions, both sides)

1. Start with your feet hip-width apart, hands by your sides and thumbs up.

2. Step forward with your left leg and bend your knee to 90 degrees. Let your back leg follow that movement.

3. As you sink into your lunge, let your arms swing upwards, beside your ears.

4. As you step back to the starting position, let your arms return to neutral. Repeat 10 times on each leg.

**Prone Slider Opener
(10 repetitions)**

1. Lie face down on the floor, with your arms out to the sides, in line with your shoulders, and both palms facing down, resting on Bodyism gliding discs. (Again, if you don't have Bodyism discs, you could use paper plates.)

2. Initiate the movement by squeezing your shoulder blades together and slightly raising your upper chest a few inches off the floor while simultaneously lowering your arms towards your sides.

3. Hold and squeeze before returning to the starting position. Repeat 10 times.

**Begging-Man Pose
(10 repetitions)**

1. Begin with feet hip-width apart, elbows bent at 90 degrees and squeezing gently at the sides of your ribcage. Place your forearms forward, with palms up and hands open. Inhale into your mid-back, pressing your shoulder blades down.

2. On the exhale, move your forearms out to the sides, keeping your elbows tucked in close to your ribs.

3. On the inhale, bring your forearms forward again, keeping your hands in front of your elbows. Feel the bottom tips of your shoulder blades squeezing towards your spine. Repeat 10 times.

**Active Leg Raise
(10 repetitions, both sides)**

1. Lie on your back, with both legs straight.

2. Pull one knee towards your chest, grasping behind the knee with both hands. Straighten your lower leg as much as possible, without letting your knee move away from your chest.

3. Hold the stretch for two seconds. Relax and return to the starting position. Complete 10 repetitions on one side before repeating with the opposite leg.

**Pigeon Stretch
(30 seconds, both sides)**

1. Slide your right knee forward, towards your right hand, keeping your foot facing toes-down on the floor.

2 Angle your right knee at two o'clock. Slide your left leg back as far as your hips will allow.

3. Keep your hips square to the floor.

4. Keeping your torso upright, reach down to steady yourself with your hands on the floor. Try to sink your hips forward and down. If you feel comfortable, you can fold forward with your torso to meet your right knee.

5. Hold for 30 seconds and return to the top. Then repeat on the other leg.

**Hug the World
(10 repetitions, both sides)**

1. Lie face up, with knees bent at 90 degrees. Roll onto your right side and squeeze your thighs together, arms out in front.

2. Keeping your bottom arm and your knees pinned to the ground, rotate your chest and top arm away, trying to place your back on the ground.

3. Extend the same arm and sweep it along the ground towards your head, until it is straight overhead, then sweep it down again behind you, towards your butt and back over to the starting position. Repeat 10 times on one side before switching legs and repeating with the opposite arm.

**Child's Pose
(1–2 minutes)**

1. Get on your hands and knees and walk your hands away, in front of you.

2. Lower your buttocks down to sit on your heels. Let your arms drag along the floor as you sit back, stretching your entire spine.

3. Once you settle onto your heels, bring your hands next to your feet and relax.

4. Breathe into your back. Rest your forehead on the floor. Hold this for a minute or two, until you feel recharged and ready to get on with the rest of your day.

SLEEP

'Sleep is medicine.'

Why is sleep a pillar of health?

Sleep is when the magic happens. It's your body's opportunity to regenerate, recharge and replenish. It's when everything you did throughout the day gets processed — physically, mentally and emotionally. Without proper, good-quality sleep, any transformation to your overall wellbeing becomes difficult or close to impossible. On the wonderful flip side of that, a good night of deep, nourishing, quality sleep has the power to transform your mind and body.

If you're exercising intelligently and eating nourishing foods but not sleeping well, it's like having lots of fuel in your car, but a flat tyre. If I don't sleep well for a few nights in a row, I spend the day slightly hysterical and things don't feel quite 'right'. I lose my sense of certainty and stability.

A good night's sleep will help you deal with the endless stream of Instagram 'bikini' and 'butt' pictures that make you want to punch your phone. It will also give your brain a much-needed chance to process all the other things going on in your life, so that you wake up the next day feeling fresh, recharged and restored.

Sleep is also the time when our body does most of its physical restoration, as well as when we actually burn fat and metabolize all of the things that need to be dealt with. What I am trying to say is this: please don't underestimate the importance of sleep! It is the foundation on which your health (both physical and mental) is built. Plus, when you're getting enough, it stops you acting like a crazy person.

The Biology of Sleep: When we sleep, our body gets to work; it's when the magic happens. Sleep enables the following changes to occur:
• Brain development
• Metabolism of fat
• Appetite regulation
• Immune strength improvement
• Increased creativity
• Memory enhancement

A 2014 study from Duke NUS Graduate Medical School found that the less we sleep, the faster our brains age. This obviously has a direct effect on our overall wellbeing. Another study, from Uppsala University in Sweden, showed that men who reported suffering sleep problems were one and a half times more likely to develop Alzheimer's (by the way, movement is another very powerful way of preventing this — look back at the Movement chapter on pages 46–73).

Sleep is closely connected with mental health. Researchers in France have found that consistently early bedtimes help to reduce our risk of mental illness. That's because sleep disturbances affect our dopamine level (a neurotransmitter associated with the 'pleasure' part of our brain), so limited sleep can be a trigger for depression, schizophrenia and bipolar disorder.

In traditional Chinese medicine, it is believed that each organ has its point of highest and lowest energy. This 24-hour cycle is thought to help us know which organs and energy channels are recharging at certain times of the night. It shows us just how vital sleep is for our body to repair optimally.

Many people make the mistake of underestimating the importance of sleep, treating it as the least essential of the four pillars. But sleep is the missing piece in the puzzle of perfect health.

Is sleep the most important pillar of all?

From the moment you wake up, if you've had a good night's sleep, you'll be more inclined to make better, kinder and more powerful food choices, and be in a better place to make decisions and react to situations in general. You'll be calmer, more centred and self-aware, and less prone to ridiculous behaviour (such as tantrums, angry outbursts and regrettable fashion statements). So, is sleep the most important pillar? It's difficult to say, because, if you don't move well and eat properly, you will, in turn, have a tough time sleeping. But, on the other hand, if you don't sleep well, then you won't move with as much energy and focus, your food choices will be poorer and your tired mental state will just make life generally more difficult to deal with. If you can really master getting a nourishing night's sleep, you'll find you feel less stressed and are more likely to be kind to yourself — both of which will feed into the way you approach the other three pillars.

What if I only 'need' a few hours sleep?

Some people supposedly function brilliantly on five hours a night. I've read stories of people like Leonardo Da Vinci and Thomas Edison (who apparently developed diabetes) and other geniuses who barely slept. But, of course, aside from their famous achievements, I do wonder how happy they truly were in their day-to-day lives. (By the way, I'm not criticizing either of these people; I'm just saying that maybe we shouldn't use them as an example of how to live a happy, healthy life... They obviously didn't have the time or energy for Pilates!)

In the past, I've been addicted to not sleeping. (Yes, that is a thing.) I went through a stage of going to bed at 2 a.m. and waking up for work at 5 a.m. My closest friend started to notice my mental state and said he was worried about me. I'd wake up in the morning almost hysterical, promising myself I'd have an early night that evening, but then the evening would come round and I'd be keeping myself busy until the early hours of the morning. I'd eventually collapse into bed completely exhausted.

And the cycle went on and on. It was only once I realized it had turned into an unhealthy habit that I decided I had to change it.

Once I'd realized how important sleep was, I set out to change my relationship with it and began go to bed at the same time (10 p.m.) as often as I could, and to wake up at the same time every morning. Within just two weeks, my unhealthy habit of staying up past bedtime had been replaced with a much healthier one.

Scientifically speaking, I had messed up my sleep pattern — better known as my 'circadian rhythm'. In human beings, the circadian rhythm is determined by a small group of brain cells located in the hypothalamus (above the optic nerve). In order for our circadian rhythm to work properly, it needs constant input in the form of natural light. For example, when the light shines through the curtains in the morning, our body will gear up, and when the sun sets in the evening, it will wind down, preparing us for sleep. However, modern technology has elbowed its unnaturally bright way in and messed up our natural clock, resulting in many of us having 'tuned out' of our own circadian rhythm and making us think that we only need a few hours' sleep, when in reality we need much more.

A study by Exeter University found that 'sleep almost doubles our chances of remembering previously unrecalled material.' If you want to be sharp and focused in the day, you need to sleep properly the night before.

And it's not just for our mental health, either, according to Dr David Gozal, chairman of paediatrics at the University of Chicago Comer Children's Hospital. He explains that 'fragmented sleep changes how the immune system deals with cancer in ways that make the disease more aggressive.' Our immune system is certain to suffer if we haven't had enough rest. Dr Axel Steiger at Munich's Max Planck Institute of Psychiatry says, 'with an infection, patients become sleepy, and [...] sleep helps them recover.' This is nature's way of trying to help us heal. But it only works if we let it.

What should I do to get a good night's sleep?

1. Make sleep a priority. By simply understanding and recognizing how important sleep is, you will start to take it a bit more seriously.

2. It's all about creating a routine, a familiar ritual that your body and brain recognize, so you can start to truly unwind and prepare for a wonderful night's rest. If you can create this ritual and stick to it, you will very soon be sleeping like a baby (and I don't mean wetting the bed and crying all night! I mean the perfect peace of baby sleep, with an angelic smile across your face).

3. If you can get hold of it, use the Bodyism supplement I created called Serenity. I spent years craving something sweet just before bed so I spent a really long time developing this supplement so that it wouldn't raise my sugar and energy levels but would help me wind down for a great night's sleep. Serenity is my desert-island item; it's made with calming herbs that help lower anxiety levels and combat the stress hormones that dump fat on your tummy. Serenity also contains hops, oats and camomile to help your body relax and promote a deep, restful, rejuvenating sleep. If you can't buy it then try and get in the habit of having a cup of camomile tea before bed and if you really want something sweet then go for a square of dark/bittersweet chocolate.

4. Try to get into bed by 10 p.m. for a 6 a.m. wake up, because eight hours is the perfect amount of sleep your body needs to achieve all the physical and mental restoration necessary during the night.

5. It may sound strange, but try to live by what I like to call 'the caveman approach'. When the sun goes down in the evening, dim the lights in your house, flat or apartment. Just as a caveman would light a fire at night, this is the modern-day equivalent. Limit the use of electronic devices in the evenings, such as phones, tablets, laptops, computers and televisions. This further reduces external stresses on your mind

and body, calming you down before bedtime, rather than stimulating you more. It might sound silly, but it does work.

If you can apply a few of these suggestions, within just a few weeks I guarantee you will feel more energetic and less anxious. (And, believe it or not, the decrease in stress can also lead to a flatter tummy, too!)

What if I get stressed about the fact I can't sleep?

While we need to understand the importance of sleep, we don't want that, in itself, to become a stressful factor. So many people have trouble with sleep and then spend hours worrying about it, which only creates more stress and just adds to the problem. Remind yourself that some of the most well-known meditation practitioners, like the Dalai Lama, purposefully wake up in the middle of the night to do two to three hours of meditation. Knowing that some of the most mindful people on the planet are up in the middle of the night helps calm me down when I'm lying there, wide awake. Think of this as time when you aren't expected to do anything, and treat it as a wonderful opportunity to meditate.

What if my to-do list is keeping me awake?

I call this 'spinning': when your mind is running through your endless to-do list and going round in circles. It's when you can't stop thinking of all the things you didn't get done that day and are stressing about all the things you need to do tomorrow. Spinning makes it impossible to calm your mind down and switch off. What you need to do is this: write it down. And I don't mean on your phone. Get a pen and a notebook, and write it all down. Promise yourself you will tick these things off tomorrow, then close your notebook and go to sleep or do your meditation.

Top Tip I learnt a great technique from my mum, which is a really simple meditation practice and can help relieve the pressure of feeling like you must go to sleep.

1. Close your eyes.
2. Focus on your breathing. Breathe into your stomach and feel it rise and fall.
3. Let your thoughts float in, and then out again.

This simple process is incredibly nourishing and way more beneficial than getting up and watching television, reading a book or answering emails. Eventually, you will drift off without even realizing it. Simply reframing the fact you are awake as an opportunity (i.e. for you to meditate without deadlines or distractions), rather than a problem, will help calm you down, enable you to enjoy meditating and inevitably drift off to sleep. Even if you are up all night doing it, that's fine! It's way more restful than anything else you could be doing. In fact, it's brilliant.

Can we eat our way to better sleep?

Not necessarily, but we can definitely eat and drink our way to a bad night's sleep (or, indeed, a lifetime of bad nights). Here are the main offenders:

Coffee. Relying on caffeine and sugar to get through the day can cause you to end up in a constant 'wired and tired' state. I love coffee, but caffeine has a powerful effect on our bodies for much longer than we think. A study from Wayne State University and Henry Ford Hospital in Detroit, Michigan, found that consuming caffeine six hours before bed can shorten sleep by as much as one hour. So our caffeine cut-off should start well before the evening.

Late-night snacks. If you eat just before bed, your body has to work hard to digest the food while you are trying to fall asleep, which can negatively affect your circadian rhythm and therefore your sleep–wake cycle. Acid reflux is also a hugely common problem. Life sometimes get in the way, so if you do have to eat late, then choose foods that contain nutrients known to promote good sleep. Foods rich in tryptophan, such as oats, beans, rice or turkey, are a good choice, as are foods that contain magnesium, such as seeds, nuts, leafy greens and bananas, as magnesium can help relax your nervous system. I try not to eat anything for at least two hours before bed and drink a cup of Bodyism Serenity supplement mixed with rice milk instead — it tastes like chocolate milk!

Alcohol. Many people believe that a drink before bed helps them sleep. Alcohol is discussed in more depth in the Nutrition chapter (see pages 33–35), so I will just mention here why alcohol does not help you sleep. A study carried out in 2015 by the University of Melbourne proved that alcohol works as a sleep disrupter. 'The quality of sleep you get is significantly altered and disrupted,' says the author of that study, Christian Nichols.

I had a client who had just returned to London from New York after 10 years. We recommended that she try the Bodyism Serenity supplement, so she swapped her nightly glass of red wine for a scoop of Serenity mixed with nut milk. She came back two weeks later and told me she'd had her best night's sleep in 10 years. She'd even got her husband to try it (he normally makes a point of not being healthy) and, 30 minutes after drinking it, he took himself off to bed, whereas normally he'd have been double-screening (on his phone and the TV) until 1 a.m. It was the first time they'd felt well-rested in years!

Do I burn fat when I sleep?

Sleep deprivation results in higher levels of stress and puts our bodies on high alert for danger. This stressed-out state leads to the release of cortisol, which in genuinely stressful situations can in fact save your life. However, when cortisol is constantly being released, it encourages your body to store fat around your stomach. That's why so many stressed-out and sleep-deprived people hold fat on their tummy.

A 2012 Harvard Medical School study found that healthy adults who normally slept an average of 8 hours and were asked to sleep an average of 5.6 hours a night for three weeks had a decreased resting metabolic rate and increased glucose levels after meals, compared to before the experiment. Both of these effects increased their risk of obesity and diabetes.

If we haven't had a good night's sleep, the next day we're much more likely to eat foods that just don't work for us. In a University of Pennsylvania study, one group of participants was kept awake all night, while another group was allowed to sleep. The people who stayed up all night ate nearly 1,000 additional calories overnight, and the next day they ate far more than the group who had slept. We know we are less decisive on little sleep (at least, I think we are, or maybe we're not... oh no, I didn't sleep well last night!), so it's easy to see why we'd choose unhealthy foods and have less self-control if we haven't had a good night's sleep. Our willpower weakens, which leads to unhealthy choices.

How can I create a routine to help me sleep?

There is no single piece of advice I can give you to help you wind down for a good night's sleep, but making good habits, which help your body and mind relax before bed, will give you every chance of getting a proper rest.

One thing I've learnt from my kids is that routines and rituals can really help. We had to teach them how to sleep, because they would lie there and just didn't know how to drift off. I remember, with my daughter, Charlotte, I had to literally close her eyes for her and then I'd stay there with her until she dropped off. Charlotte and Leo have a bedtime routine which starts way before bedtime. Their 'winding down' time includes a bath, a story we read from a book and a 'nisery' (that's what Charlotte calls my made-up stories), and then we put them into bed and they go to sleep. Rituals like this are just as useful for us as adults; we just need to find our own individual winding-down routine to get our mind and body ready for sleep.

So how should we do it? I start winding down once I've put the kids to bed. Chrissy and I will eat dinner together, then we'll usually do another hour of work before catching up on an episode of a boxset. We'll then switch off the TV, go to the bedroom and we always put our phones in another room (more on this below) and then, finally, I'll have a cup of Serenity, get into bed and, as I go to sleep, I focus on what I'm grateful for.

Despite this, I have to confess that late nights are still my vice. Every few weeks I'll still have a night where Chrissy goes to bed, but I just stay up, scrolling through my phone and watching TV, and it won't be until I'm completely exhausted that I make myself go to bed. I always feel terrible the next day. So, even while writing about the importance of this pillar, the truth is I'm still struggling to get to grips with it myself.

Why should I write a gratitude journal?

Chrissy and I have made writing a gratitude list an important part of our bedtime routine. Focusing on gratitude and being in a state of gratitude is one of the most powerful states of being. The very fact that you are grateful means something great has happened. So, finding time to be grateful is one of the best things you can do for your entire wellbeing. Think about how you feel when you are genuinely grateful. Now imagine feeling that way every minute of every day. Of course, in reality, we can't stay entirely grateful all day long, but if we can actively think of something we're genuinely grateful for, it can really help unwind the stress that has built up from the day.

For most people, it won't be, 'I am grateful for the sunshine,' or, 'I am grateful for the cool breeze,' (though, great, if it is). For most people, it's more likely to be something like finding a toilet when you were busting for a wee (I can say that because we're friends now — and there are very few things that make you feel as intensely grateful as this!) or having a glass of water when you were really thirsty.

I find that my gratitude journal focuses my mind on the blessings in my life, rather than on the list of things that might stress me out. Arianna Huffington wrote about this perfectly in her book, *The Sleep Revolution*. She explains, 'it's the stresses and setbacks that seem to take centre stage in our minds once our head hits the pillow. They are the preening, attention-seeking, spotlight-hogging divas of our bedtime hours, ignoring the stage manager begging them to exit. A gratitude list is a great way to knock them down a peg, shift the spotlight and make sure our blessings get the closing scene of the night.'

Focus on that feeling of gratitude and try to let it consume you before you go to bed. Reserve five minutes every night for thinking about what you are truly grateful for. You can write it down (I love *The Five-Minute Journal* by Intelligent Change, which you can buy online worldwide), say it out loud or simply say it in your head. I encourage you to fully express yourself and feel fine about doing so. There is nothing to be afraid of or embarrassed about. Let yourself go. What you're grateful for will change every day. Be curious and find gratitude in even the smallest of things.

Here are some things on my gratitude list:

I am grateful for my healthy body.
I am grateful for the food that I ate today.
I am grateful for the hugs that I got from my children and wife.
I am grateful that I have a home — a warm place to live in.

What's the most powerful way to start the day?

Those first few moments at the start of each day are your most powerful. Think of what you can do today to elevate it beyond yesterday. Who can you be?

Before you get up and start your day, remind yourself how powerful you are. You can do this by finding a mantra, which you can say out loud, write down or say in your head. It should be something which reminds you that you have the courage, kindness, intelligence, power and strength to change everything.

Find words that function as your driving force, that give you your power and purpose, and that define who you are. Find words that inspire you and leave no room for pettiness, jealousy or revenge.

Here are some you might like to try:

I am kind.
I am intelligent.
I am loving.
I am inspiring.

So much of our day is consumed with obsessing over details, which then leads to stress, but if you remind yourself of the greater and more important affirmations, then everything else will take care of itself. There's no way we can predict all the things that we might be faced with throughout the day, but we can remind ourselves to be loving, kind, strong and great. It will put you in a far more powerful place to deal with whatever comes your way each day. Be the manifestation of those things. That is very powerful.

Is meditation important?

There is so much in this world that we don't know or understand. Our awareness only allows us to see so much and we can only see what we can comprehend. If all we are doing is focusing on our job, our appearance, our income and our relationships, then we are asleep to our own deeper dimensions. Meditation and sleep are like brain retreats, allowing us to achieve a stillness that is available to all of us, if we choose to reach for it. Meditation nourishes and unwinds the mind and body, which is not only beneficial for us individually, but also for those around us. For me, meditation is like having a massage for the soul. A 2009 Stanford study showed that a six-week meditation course helped people who had trouble sleeping to fall asleep twice as quickly. The science proves it: meditation helps us sleep, and together the two can totally transform our overall wellbeing.

The Roman emperor Marcus Aurelius wrote in his book *Meditations*, 'People look for retreats for themselves, in the country, by the coast or in the hills, when it's possible to retreat into yourself any time you want. There is nowhere that a person can find a more peaceful or trouble-free retreat than in his own mind.' Meditation doesn't mean you have to become a monk on top of a mountain; it's just about dedicating time to yourself when you can focus on your breath and let your thoughts float in and out. There is no 'one way' to meditate and these days there are endless apps, books and courses to help you find what's right for you.

Can I afford not to meditate?

I had a conversation about this with a great friend who I deeply admire; he has meditated for many years and found great positives from it. Over time, he's learnt to take that feeling he got from practising meditation and fuse it into his daily life. So, rather than experiencing 'Stress-stress-stress-stress. Pause for meditation. Stress-stress-stress,' he has now found a way to feel genuinely happy and peaceful all day long and integrate the benefits of meditation into every minute of every day. I try to do that in my life, too. Meditation is amazing, but rather than relying on it for downtime, try and inject that ease you get from meditation into your everyday life, into every minute of every day, until it becomes part of who you actually are.

Eventually, your whole life should be a meditation on happiness, joy, courage, kindness and all of the things that are important to you.

How can I relax to recharge?

Being relaxed doesn't have to mean that you're sleepy or lazy or not getting things done. For instance, in a tennis match, the player who wins the tournament is the one who stays calm and focused. It's the same with fighting (one of the most stressful situations you could put yourself in, with not one moment when you can afford to be lazy — otherwise, you lose): the fighter who can relax through it, remaining calm and serene, is usually the winner. That's what I've learnt from jiu-jitsu. It's like quicksand — the more you struggle and stress, the more difficult the situation becomes, while having a sense of ease and learning to truly relax is the way to win. It's like being in *The Matrix*! When I fight against someone who isn't as relaxed as I am, that's when I win. I'm not naturally talented or a phenomenal athlete, but I win competitions because I can stay calm. It's the same in your everyday life. Some people don't feel they are working hard unless they are stressed, and they fear people won't respect what they say unless they deliver it in a 'shouty', stressed-out, urgent way — but it's just not true. People respond best to calmness, and it shines through. Finding peace in the chaos is true mastery and yet so achievable.

Remember the words of one of my favourite poems: *If* by Rudyard Kipling.

> If you can keep your head when all about you
> Are losing theirs and blaming it on you,
> If you can trust yourself when all men doubt you,
> But make allowance for their doubting too;
> If you can wait and not be tired by waiting,
> [...]
> Yours is the Earth and everything that's in it,
> And — which is more — you'll be a Man, my son!

Bodyism Meditations

Here are some meditations for you to add to your morning, day or winding-down routine:

On-the-Go Meditation

This is one to practise when you are out and about. Sometimes we just need a few minutes to reset and this meditation will do exactly that.

Focus on all your senses, with no judgement.

Be completely present to where you are. Notice the colour of the trees, the wind in your face, the smells surrounding you and the feeling of your feet in your shoes. Rather than judge, notice the sensations and be present in that very moment. Any thoughts that drop in, accept them and let them pass.

Be in the present moment, right here, right now.

Power of the Breath Meditation

Always come back to the power of your breath; it can totally transform your mental and physical wellbeing. Full, deep breathing can lower tension and stress, and will help you totally relax.

The object of this meditation is to learn how to really get in touch with the rhythm of your breathing and learn to breathe in a relaxed, unstressed way. It can be practised in any position, but it's best to start off by lying on your back, with your knees bent.

This meditation can be practised daily, either first thing, or as part of your winding-down routine. You can do it almost anywhere; it's a relaxation tool which you can use any time you need it.

Caution: Some people get dizzy the first few times they practise this, but it's just your body adjusting.

Place one hand on your stomach and your other hand on your chest. Notice how your hands move as you breathe in and out.

Practise breathing so that the hand on your tummy rises when you inhale and the hand on your chest stays still. Inhale for five seconds through your nose, pause for three seconds, and exhale for five seconds through your mouth. Keep your shoulders relaxed throughout.

When you have noticed your stomach rising and falling a few times, add the second step to your breathing: inhale first into your stomach, and then continue inhaling into your chest. You should feel the hand on your chest rising, too.

As you exhale, feel the tension leaving your body as you become more and more relaxed.

Practise this for five minutes. Notice the constant movement of your breathing, like waves coming in and out.

Recharge Meditation

This is a great meditation to do first thing. It always energizes me for the day ahead; make it a habit.

Begin in a comfortable seated position, with your spine supported and your palms resting, either face-up or down, on your knees. (If you can't sit on the floor, a chair is fine, or even lying down is okay — as long as the spine is straight.)

Turn your attention to your breath. Notice your inhalation and exhalation.

What is the rhythm of your breathing? A stressed state will often cause a faster inhalation and an unfulfilled exhalation. A slow and calm exhalation stimulates the parasympathetic nervous system, increasing your ability to digest and detoxify. It is also on the exhalation that we release toxins in the form of carbon dioxide.

Every breath you take is recharging you. Start to count with each breath.

Inhale for three seconds. Hold it for three seconds. Exhale for six seconds.

Repeat for eight rounds — simply count the rounds on your hand by touching your thumb to each finger as you move to the next one.

At the top of each inhalation, in your head repeat the mantra, 'I am recharged', and, on each exhalation, visualize all the toxins and tensions leaving your body.

Notice how you feel after these lengthened breaths.

Slowly open your eyes.

Relaxed Meditation

We do not become stronger, fitter or leaner when we train; instead, the transformation actually happens when we relax. If we can't relax, our training and nutritious diet will not be supported by the body. This meditation is about relaxation.

Begin in a comfortable seated position, with your spine supported and palms resting, either face-up or down, on your knees. (If you can't sit on the floor, a chair or lying down is fine too — as long as the spine is straight.)

Turn your attention to your breath. Notice your inhalation and exhalation. What is the rhythm of your breathing? Relax your body by lengthening the breath.

Every breath you take is relaxing you. Start to count with each breath.

Inhale for three seconds. Hold it for three seconds. Exhale for six seconds.

Repeat for eight rounds, counting the rounds on your hand by touching your thumb to each finger as you go.

Once you have relaxed the body, repeat this mantra in synchronization with your breath:

Inhale: 'I am.'

Exhale: 'relaxed.'

Repeat three times.

Open your eyes slowly. Take a moment to notice the connection between your body and mind.

Your Unique Meditation

This time, you have the opportunity to choose your own mantra. Choose a mantra that suits your current life situation. Think of what your body, mind and spirit need most and affirm it with your mantra and breath. Add this into your day whenever you need to refocus, or when you just need some extra support.

Begin in a comfortable seated position, with your spine supported and palms resting, either face-up or down, on your knees. (Again, if you can't sit on the floor, a chair or even lying down is fine — as long as the spine is straight.)

Turn your attention to your breath. Notice your inhalation and exhalation. What is the rhythm of your breathing?

Every breath you take is cleansing you. Start to count with each breath.

Inhale for three seconds. Hold it for three seconds. Exhale for six seconds.

Repeat for three rounds — counting the rounds, as before, by touching your thumb to each finger as you move to the next one. Once you have relaxed your body, repeat the mantra of your choice in synchronization with your breath:

Inhale: 'I am.'

Exhale: 'Happy' / 'Calm' / 'Free' / 'Open' / 'Organized' / 'Capable' / 'Beautiful' / 'Energized'... (The choice is yours.)

Connect to the feeling of that particular affirmation and let it fill you with eagerness for your life.

Repeat eight times.

Open your eyes slowly. Take a moment to notice the connection to your body and mind.

Did You Know? An entire industry has been created to fuel a population who are living with continuous exhaustion. In the US, more than 55 million prescriptions for sleeping pills were written in 2014 alone, with sales exceeding a billion dollars. Jerome Siegel, director of UCLA's Centre for Sleep Research, explained that, in the near future, 'people will look back on the sleeping-pill era as we now look back on the acceptance of cigarette smoking.' The chronic use of sleeping pills is a total disaster. The amount of money, time and brainpower that goes into them is not solving any problems. These pills do not offer a magic solution to giving us a good night's sleep; they just distract us from the benefits of real, restorative sleep.

Here are just some of the side effects of the sleeping tablets sold worldwide: anxiety; bladder pain; bloody or cloudy urine; change in walking and balance; chills; cold sweats; cough; crying; decreased awareness or responsiveness; delusions; dementia; depersonalization; dizziness; dry mouth; dysphoria; euphoria; fainting; frequent urge to urinate; hyperventilation; irregular heartbeats; irritability; light-headedness when getting up from a lying or sitting position; lower back or side pain; painful urination (burning, itching, numbness, prickling); paranoia, 'pins and needles'; rapidly changing moods; severe sleepiness; shakiness in the legs, arms, hands or feet; shortness of breath; violent behaviours.

A study from the Scripps Research Institute, led by Dr Daniel Kripke, found that those who had taken 18 sleeping tablets in a year had a risk of death three times higher during the two-and-half-year study than those who had not taken any pills. I could also write an endless list of the links between disease and sleeping pills. They're linked to cancer, infertility, dementia, the list goes on. Reaching for a sleeping tablet is the opposite of being kind to yourself.

BODYISM TWO-WEEK BLUEPRINT

This is your opportunity to elevate your health and create a beautiful, vibrant and energized body. When you embrace this Blueprint, you will begin to learn the many different ways in which your body is speaking to you. You can let go of old, unhealthy and unhelpful habits. Once you have mastered the art of listening to your body, you will never need another diet book, exercise plan, app or any other 'guide' again because the answers will come from the only expert you will ever need — you. This is the first step you can make to 'Be Kind To Yourself'.

WEEK ONE

Monday

Mindset: Say your affirmations and choose one meditation to fit into your day.

Movement: Prehab Circuit, 2x Perfect Posture Circuit, Quick Cardio Burst, 2x Perky Butt Circuit, Quick Cardio Burst, Regenerate Circuit

A Powerful Action: Drink two litres of water/herbal tea throughout your day.

Nutrition: Breakfast — The Protein Wrap
Lunch — Bowl of your choice
Shake — Body Brilliance Shake
Dinner — Courgette Lasagne

Sleep: Write/think/speak aloud your gratitude journal (see page 82). Please try to be winding down by 10 p.m.

Tuesday

Mindset: Say your affirmations and choose one meditation to fit into your day.

Movement: Prehab Circuit, 2x Long Lean Legs, Quick Cardio Burst, 2x Flat-tummy Circuit, Quick Cardio Burst, Regenerate Circuit

A Powerful Action: Remember to chew your food.

Nutrition: Breakfast — Simply Granola, with nut milk and a sprinkling of berries
Lunch — Alkalizing Supergreen Soup, with a side of your choice
Shake — Beauty Food Shake
Dinner — Turmeric Dhal, with some greens

Sleep: Write/think/speak aloud your gratitude journal (see page 82). Please try to be winding down by 10 p.m.

Wednesday

Mindset: Say your affirmations and choose one meditation to fit into your day.

Movement: 30-minute walk/yoga class/try a new class with a friend.

A Powerful Action: Remember to add a portion of greens to one of your meals today.

Nutrition: Breakfast — The Egg Bowl.
Lunch — Bowl of your choice
Shake — Berry Burn Shake
Dinner — Poached Coconut Chicken and Cauli-rice, with greens (make extra chicken for tomorrow)

Sleep: Write/think/speak aloud your gratitude journal (see page 82). Please try to be winding down by 10 p.m.

Thursday

Mindset: Say your affirmations and choose one meditation to fit into your day.

Movement: Prehab Circuit, 2x Perky Butt Circuit, Quick Cardio Burst, 2x Long Lean Legs, Quick Cardio Burst, Regenerate Circuit

A Powerful Action: Do a random act of kindness today; it's the best way to create power in your own life.

Nutrition: Breakfast — The Protein Wrap
Lunch — Leftover Coconut Chicken, with Kabbouleh
Shake — Ultimate Clean Shake
Dinner — Ultimate Fish Pie, with greens

Sleep: Write/think/speak aloud your gratitude journal (see page 82). Please try to be winding down by 10 p.m.

Friday

Mindset: Say your affirmations and choose one meditation to fit into your day.

Movement: Prehab Circuit, 2x Perfect Posture Circuit, Quick Cardio Burst, 2x Flat-tummy Circuit, Quick Cardio Burst, Regenerate Circuit

A Powerful Action: Commit to switching your phone off at 9 p.m. tonight.

Nutrition: Breakfast — Bircher Muesli
Lunch — Bowl of your choice
Shake — Chai Cashew Mylk
Dinner — Keralan Fish Curry, with veg of your choice

Sleep: Write/think/speak aloud your gratitude journal (see page 82). Please try to be winding down by 10 p.m.

Saturday

Mindset: Say your affirmations and choose one meditation to fit into your day.

Movement: Prehab Circuit, 2x Perky Butt Circuit, Quick Cardio Burst, 2x Flat-tummy Circuit, Quick Cardio Burst, Regenerate Circuit

A Powerful Action: This may sound corny but it's one of the most powerful things you can do... Tell someone you love them today.

Nutrition: Breakfast — Brunchy Baked Eggs
Lunch — Chickpea Dosa Wrap
Shake — Body Brilliance Shake
Dinner — Perfect Roast Chicken, with a side of your choice and some greens

Sleep: Write/think/speak aloud your gratitude journal (see page 82). Please try to be winding down by 10 p.m.

Sunday

Mindset: Say your affirmations and choose one meditation to fit into your day.

Movement: Rest and try to get a massage.

A Powerful Action: Remember to chill today.

Nutrition: Breakfast — Buckwheat, Egg, Carrot and Mushroom Crêpes
Lunch — Turmeric, Sweet Potato, Ginger and Coconut Soup, with buckwheat and radish salad
Snack — Bodyism Cookie (remember portion control, here — you can always have cookies again)
Dinner — Bodyism Frittata (make enough for breakfast tomorrow)

Sleep: Write/think/speak aloud your gratitude journal (see page 82). Please try to be winding down by 10 p.m.

Tuesday

Mindset: Say your affirmations and choose one meditation to fit into your day.

Movement: Prehab Circuit, 2x Perfect Posture Circuit, Quick Cardio Burst, 2x Perky Butt Circuit, Quick Cardio Burst, Regenerate Circuit

A Powerful Action: Say thank you... It's the fastest way to get yourself into a state of gratitude, which is one of the happiest, most wonderful states of being.

Nutrition: Breakfast — Three-Grain Porridge
Lunch — Chicken Pho
Shake — Ultimate Clean Shake
Dinner — Tuna Poke Bowl

Sleep: Write/think/speak aloud your gratitude journal (see page 82). Please try to be winding down by 10 p.m.

WEEK TWO

Monday

Mindset: Say your affirmations and choose one meditation to fit into your day.

Movement: Prehab Circuit, 2x Perfect Posture Circuit, Quick Cardio Burst, 2x Long Lean Legs, Quick Cardio Burst, Regenerate Circuit

A Powerful Action: Spend five minutes focusing on your breath.

Nutrition: Breakfast — Leftover Bodyism Frittata
Lunch — Bowl of your choice
Shake — Body Brilliance Shake
Dinner — Perfect Roast Chicken, with a side of your choice (make sure you cook enough chicken so you'll have leftovers)

Sleep: Write/think/speak aloud your gratitude journal (see page 82). Please try to be winding down by 10 p.m.

Wednesday

Mindset: Say your affirmations and choose one meditation to fit into your day.

Movement: 30-minute walk/a dance class/a boxing class — try something new!

A Powerful Action: Drink two litres of water/herbal tea throughout your day.

Nutrition: Breakfast — Açai Bowl
Lunch — Bowl of your choice
Shake — Beauty Food Shake
Dinner — Turmeric Dhal (make enough for tomorrow)

Sleep: Write/think/speak aloud your gratitude journal (see page 82). Please try to be winding down by 10 p.m.

Thursday

Mindset: Say your affirmations and choose one meditation to fit into your day.

Movement: Prehab Circuit, 2x Flat-tummy Circuit, Quick Cardio Burst, 2x Long Lean Legs, Quick Cardio Burst, Regenerate Circuit

A Powerful Action: Choose to be more powerful than all of your excuses.

Nutrition: Breakfast — Leftover Turmeric Dhal, with a fried egg on top!
Lunch — Alkalizing Supergreen Soup
Shake — Berry Burn Shake
Dinner — Sexy Stir-Fry, with a protein of your choice (chicken, lamb, fish)

Sleep: Write/think/speak aloud your gratitude journal (see page 82). Please try to be winding down by 10 p.m.

Friday

Mindset: Say your affirmations and choose one meditation to fit into your day.

Movement: Prehab Circuit, 2x Perfect Posture Circuit, Quick Cardio Burst, 2x Flat-tummy Circuit, Quick Cardio Burst, Regenerate Circuit

A Powerful Action: Remind yourself of your 'why', if you are tempted to fall back into old habits.

Nutrition: Breakfast — Bircher Muesli
Lunch — Bowl of your choice
Shake — Body Brilliance Shake
Dinner — Moroccan Tagine (make enough for tomorrow)

Sleep: Write/think/speak aloud your gratitude journal (see page 82). Please try to be winding down by 10 p.m.

Saturday

Mindset: Say your affirmations and choose one meditation to fit into your day.

Movement: Prehab Circuit, 2x Perky Butt Circuit, Quick Cardio Burst, 2x Flat-tummy Circuit, Quick Cardio Burst, Regenerate Circuit

A Powerful Action: Practise being present; have a conversation with someone, don't have your phone anywhere near, and listen genuinely to them.

Nutrition: Breakfast — Indian Spiced Eggs
Lunch — Turmeric, Sweet Potato, Ginger and Coconut Soup, with buckwheat and radish salad
Shake — Beauty Food Shake
Dinner — Leftover Moroccan Tagine

Sleep: Write/think/speak aloud your gratitude journal (see page 82). Please try to be winding down by 10 p.m.

Sunday

Mindset: Say your affirmations and choose one meditation to fit into your day.

Movement: Rest and try to get a massage.

A Powerful Action: Be proud of yourself, enjoy the moment, take on the lessons from your body and your experience from the past two weeks and allow them to strengthen you for the future.

Nutrition: Breakfast — Chocolate Soup (it's Sunday!)
Lunch — Miso Prawn and Aubergine Salad, and a slice of Honey Cake!
Shake — Chai Cashew Mylk
Dinner — The Perfect Burger and Sweet Potato Wedges (add some greens, please)

Sleep: Write/think/speak aloud your gratitude journal (see page 82). Please try to be winding down by 10 p.m.

THE
RECIPES

BREAKFAST

AÇAI BOWL

Our cafe in Notting Hill is becoming famous for the açai bowls we serve. Açai is one of the most nutritious fruits in the world. We blend ours with one of the Bodyism supplements to increase the protein content in each bowl and to make it even more delicious.

Our açai supplier, Rayder, is an activist for preventing deforestation in the Amazon and açai is one of the only no-timber products to come from the rainforest. So, make sure you choose high-quality frozen açai (you can find it in health stores or online) and feel proud that you are helping to save the planet and looking after your body, too. If you don't have the Bodyism supplements, substitute them for a tablespoon of hemp seeds.

serves 2

100 g/3½ oz frozen açai pulp
half a frozen banana
1 scoop Bodyism Body Brilliance or Bodyism
    Protein Excellence
50 ml/1¾ fl oz/¼ cup almond milk
75 g/2⅔ oz/½ cup frozen mixed berries

for the toppings
2 tbsp almond butter
2 tbsp Simply Granola (see page 102)
2 tbsp fresh berries
any other superfood you'd like: goji berries,
    hemp seeds, bee pollen, coconut flakes,
    chia seeds!

1. Put the açai, banana, Bodyism supplement and almond milk into a blender. Whizz it up until all the açai is mixed (if there are any unblended pieces left, then add more almond milk).

2. Spoon into bowls. Add the toppings equally into each bowl. Start with the almond butter, then granola and finally sprinkle with berries and any other superfood you want!

Top Tip Texture is everything. Aim for an ice-cream consistency, not a smoothie — it is an art!

CHOCOLATE SOUP

Otherwise known as 'Soup of Eternal Blissful Love'. I fell in love with Chrissy while eating a chocolate soup, so now I've come up with a healthy version that nourishes your body, helps you burn fat and guarantees that you will fall in love with the first person you see after eating it... It's a delicious nutrient boost for both your body and your taste buds.

If you don't have the Bodyism supplements, get them! Or, if not, then add in a tablespoon of hemp seeds to get an extra boost of protein.

---

serves 2
500 ml/17 fl oz/2 cups unsweetened
   almond milk
120 ml/4¼ fl oz/½ cup coconut yoghurt
½ tsp vanilla extract
2 bananas, frozen
3 tbsp cacao powder
3 tbsp hazelnut butter (or another nut butter
   of your choice)
handful of frozen spinach
1 scoop Bodyism Protein Excellence
   (optional)
1 scoop Bodyism Body Brilliance (optional)

for the toppings (per serving)
1 tbsp cacao nibs
1 tbsp Simply Granola (see page 102)
1 tsp hazelnut butter
1 tbsp hemp seeds
6 frozen cherries
1 tbsp coconut milk (drizzled on the top)

1. Put all the ingredients into a blender and whizz until smooth.

2. Add any topping you like!

Top Tip This also tastes delicious frozen — it is the Bodyism version of chocolate ice-cream!

THREE-GRAIN PORRIDGE

If you can, try to soak the grains for this recipe overnight. Soaking them makes them easier to digest (and quicker to cook in the morning).

serves 2

25 g/1 oz/¼ cup rolled gluten-free oats
15 g/½ oz buckwheat flakes
10 g/⅓ oz buckwheat groats
200 ml/7 fl oz/¾ cup water
100 ml/3½ fl oz almond milk
1 tbsp chia seeds
generous pinch of salt
1 tsp ground cinnamon
1 scoop Bodyism Protein Excellence

for the toppings

2 tbsp coconut yoghurt
100 g/3½ oz sugar-free strawberry jam
2 tbsp almond flakes, toasted
2 tbsp blueberries

1. Soak the oats, buckwheat flakes and groats in water overnight. Use just enough water to cover the grains.

2. Put the soaked grains, water and almond milk in a saucepan. Add the chia seeds and stir. Bring slowly to the boil. Turn down the heat and add the salt, cinnamon and Protein Excellence. Stir well until you achieve the consistency you are after.

3. Divide between two bowls, add a spoon of coconut yoghurt and strawberry jam to each, then sprinkle with almond flakes and blueberries and enjoy!

Top Tip My little boy, Leo, loves a chocolate version. Add in a scoop of Body Brilliance, one teaspoon of almond butter and one teaspoon of cacao.

BIRCHER MUESLI

This is such a wholesome breakfast and is always one of my go-to recipes in the winter months when I'm craving something that is going to keep me feeling full up till lunch. I love to mix the Bodyism Protein Excellence supplement into this recipe and eat it straight after a morning workout. Feel free to experiment with the flavour — try adding cacao or ginger, or swap the fruit for whatever is in season.

serves 2

45 g/1½ oz/½ cup rolled oats
90 g/3¼ oz/½ cup cooked quinoa
1 tbsp chia seeds
1 tbsp sunflower seeds
2 tbsp shredded coconut
1 tbsp goji berries
½ tsp ground cinnamon
½ tsp ground ginger
1 tsp vanilla extract
50 g/1¾ oz/½ cup blueberries
120 ml/4¼ fl oz/½ cup coconut water
60 ml/2 fl oz/¼ cup coconut milk
120 ml/4¼ fl oz/½ cup coconut yoghurt
1 scoop Bodyism Protein Excellence
   (optional)

for the topping

120 ml/4¼ fl oz/½ cup coconut yoghurt
handful of blueberries or stewed apple
handful of toasted coconut flakes
handful of toasted pistachio nuts, shelled
drizzle of maple syrup (optional)

1. In a bowl, mix the oats, cooked quinoa, chia seeds, sunflower seeds, shredded coconut, goji berries, cinnamon, ginger and vanilla extract.

2. In a small bowl, mash the blueberries slightly so they release their delicious juice and then stir them into the muesli.

3. Add the coconut water, milk and yoghurt and stir well. If you are adding the supplement, stir it in here too. Stir to combine well, cover, and leave in the fridge overnight.

4. In the morning, divide the mixture into two bowls. Top with a spoon of coconut yoghurt, berries or stewed apple, some coconut flakes, pistachios and, if you'd like, a small drizzle of maple syrup.

Top Tip Double the recipe and keep the mixture in a jar, so that you have a delicious quick breakfast for the week.

SIMPLY GRANOLA

Granola is often the 'Mean Girls' of breakfast. It's basically pretending to be your friend, but actually it's making you fat. Store-bought granola is so often full of sugar in all its different forms — whether it's dates or brown-rice syrup — whatever it is, it will be hidden in there. This granola is genuinely healthy and can be eaten regularly with love and joy.

serves 6

250 g/10 oz/3 cups rolled oats
250 g/8¾ oz/2 cups buckwheat flakes
50 g/1¾ oz/⅓ cup buckwheat groats
30 g/1 oz/¼ cup pecans, chopped
30 g/1 oz/¼ cup cashews (or a nut of your choice), chopped
20 g/¾ oz/¼ cup pumpkin seeds
15 g/½ oz/⅛ cup sunflower seeds
2 tbsp linseeds/flaxseeds
30 g/1 oz/½ cup coconut flakes
4 tbsp coconut oil
2 tbsp ground cinnamon
3 tsp vanilla powder
1 tsp Himalayan pink salt

1. Preheat the oven to 190°C/375°F/gas mark 5 and line 2 baking trays with parchment paper.

2. Put the oats, buckwheat flakes and groats, nuts, seeds and coconut into a big mixing bowl. Mix well.

3. In a saucepan, melt the coconut oil. Take the oil off the heat and add the cinnamon, vanilla and salt. Mix well.

4. Pour the oil mixture into the mixing bowl and stir well.

5. Spread the mixture evenly on the baking trays. Using a spatula, push the mixture firmly onto the tray. Bake for 20 minutes in the preheated oven, using the spatula to turn the granola mixture over halfway through baking.

6. Leave to cool in the baking trays. Once at room temperature, pour the granola into an airtight container. Enjoy this with rice milk or coconut yoghurt for breakfast, or sprinkle over Chocolate Soup (see page 99) or Açai Bowl (see page 96).

Top Tip Remember the granola will continue to cook once it's out of the oven so don't let it burn!

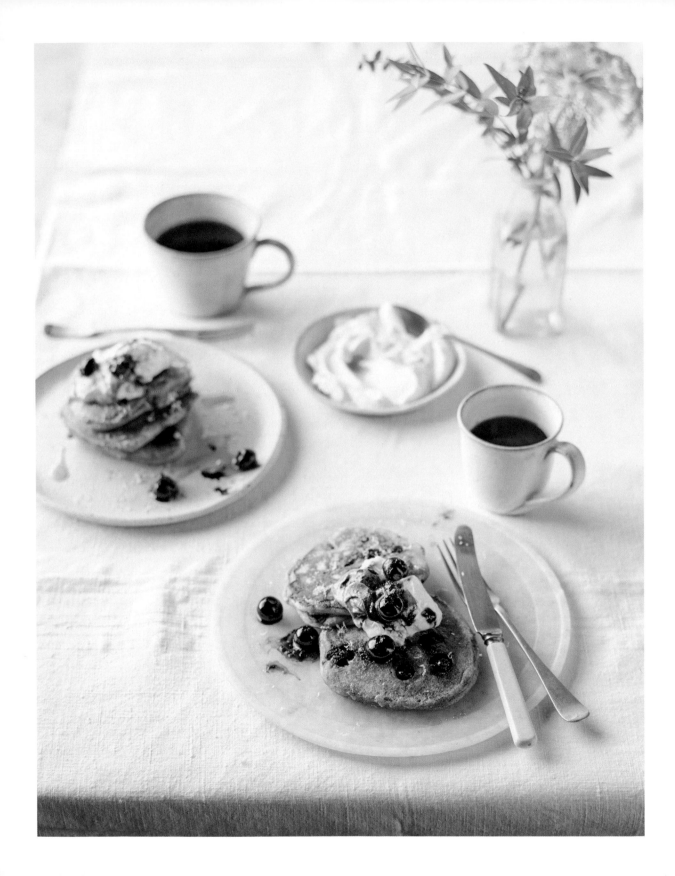

PROTEIN PANCAKES

This pancake is too legit to quit. It's an OG (original gangsta) of the Bodyism
world. Delicious and loved by everyone — children, grumpy husbands — and,
if you don't tell anyone it's healthy, they'll just keep asking for more..

serves 2 (makes a stack of 6)
1 banana, sliced
2 organic, free-range eggs
1¾ scoops Bodyism Protein Excellence
pinch of ground cinnamon
¼ tsp bicarbonate of soda/baking soda
zest of 1 lemon
2 tbsp almond milk
1 tsp coconut oil
handful of blueberries (optional)

for the toppings
4 tbsp coconut yoghurt
1 tsp almond butter
2 tbsp fresh berries

1. Put the banana, eggs, Protein Excellence, cinnamon,
   bicarbonate of soda/baking soda, lemon zest and
   almond milk into a blender. Blend it up until it is well
   mixed.

2. Add the oil to a frying pan/skillet and place over
   a medium heat, spreading the oil around the pan.

3. Add 2 tablespoons of pancake batter into the pan.
   Sprinkle with blueberries if you like. Leave to cook
   for 1–2 minutes before flipping and then cook for
   another 1–2 minutes on the other side. Do this until
   all the mixture is used up.

4. Stack the pancakes and top with coconut yoghurt,
   almond butter and fresh berries.

CHAI CARROT CHEW-CHEW

This is traditionally an Indian pudding; however, I think it makes an impressive
grain-free breakfast. You'll notice ghee enhances the sweetness of the carrots.

serves 2
2 large carrots
2 tsp coconut oil or ghee
200 ml/7 fl oz/¾ cup coconut milk
1 tbsp sultanas/golden raisins
1 tsp ground cardamom
1 tsp ground cinnamon
handful of pistachios, roughly chopped
1 tbsp chia seeds

1. Start by washing and coarsely grating the carrots,
   then set aside.

2. Heat 2 teaspoons of oil in a small saucepan over
   a low heat and add the grated carrots. Cook for
   5 minutes, until the carrots smell fragrant.

3. Add the milk, sultanas/golden raisins, cardamom
   and cinnamon and stir over a low heat for 10 minutes,
   or until the liquid is absorbed. Serve with the
   chopped pistachios and chia seeds.

ALMOND AND COCONUT PANCAKES WITH ROASTED, SPICED PEACHES

This is mouth-wateringly good — and, what's more, it's not rammed with refined sugar, chemicals, salt or any of the other junk that makes you feel less than what you deserve. There is honey in it, so don't have it every day, but when you do, enjoy it.

serves 4
for the peaches
12 peaches
1 tsp mixed spice/pumpkin pie spice
1 tsp ground ginger
1 tbsp organic honey (optional)
1 tsp grated orange zest
2 tbsp orange juice

for the pancakes
25 g/1 oz/¼ cup coconut flour
100 g/3½ oz/1 cup ground almonds
1 scoop Bodyism Protein Excellence
  (optional)
1 tsp ground ginger
1 tsp ground cinnamon
1½ tsp baking powder
4 organic, free-range eggs
200 ml/7 fl oz/¾ cup coconut milk
1 tsp vanilla extract
1 tbsp maple syrup (optional)
2 tbsp coconut oil

1. Preheat the oven to 180°C/350°F/gas mark 4 and line a baking tray with parchment paper.

2. Cut the peaches into quarters, discarding the stones.

3. Mix together the mixed spice, ginger, honey, orange zest and juice. Place two thirds of the peach quarters on the baking tray and drizzle the liquid over them.

4. Roast for 15 minutes in the preheated oven and then leave to cool. Place the cooked peaches in a bowl, reserving the juice in a separate bowl.

5. Place the remaining uncooked peaches and the juice from the cooked peaches in a food processor and blend. Pour into a small bowl and set aside.

6. To make the pancakes, mix the flour, ground almonds, Protein Excellence, ground ginger, cinnamon and baking powder in a large bowl. In a separate bowl, mix the eggs, coconut milk, vanilla extract and maple syrup (if using) together. Slowly beat this into the dry mixture to make a lovely batter.

7. Set a small non-stick frying pan/skillet over a medium heat. Add the oil and, once melted, drop a large spoonful of pancake batter into the hot pan, spreading it around the base. Cook for 1 minute, then flip and cook until golden brown. Using a spatula, lift out of the pan and set aside until all 4 pancakes are cooked.

8. Reheat the peaches and serve on top of the pancakes with a drizzle of the sauce.

INDIAN SPICED EGGS

If you're feeling adventurous and want to spice up your scrambled eggs, this is the recipe for you. Turmeric is an incredible anti-inflammatory, so not only is this delicious, but it's really good for your health, too.

serves 4

1 tbsp coconut oil
1 small red onion, finely chopped
2 garlic cloves, crushed
1 green chilli, deseeded and finely chopped
¼ tsp ground cumin
¼ tsp garam masala
¼ tsp ground turmeric
4 big tomatoes, deseeded and finely chopped
8 organic, free-range eggs, beaten
good pinch of salt and pepper
1 tbsp fresh coriander/cilantro, finely chopped (plus extra for serving)

1. Heat a large frying pan/skillet over a low to medium heat and add the oil. Fry the onion, garlic and chilli until the onion is soft (approximately 5 minutes). Add the spices and stir for another 1–2 minutes.

2. Add the tomatoes to the pan and stir. Leave to sauté for 30 seconds.

3. Pour in the eggs and lower the heat. Season with salt and pepper. Stir slowly to scramble the eggs as they cook. Remove from the heat when they are still a little runny and then stir in the coriander/cilantro. Continue to stir for another minute.

4. Serve with a Chickpea Dosa Wrap (see page 133) or a slice of sourdough toast. Garnish with a sprig of coriander/cilantro before serving.

Did You Know? Turmeric only becomes a superhero antioxidant when it is activated with pepper.

THE PROTEIN WRAP

This wrap is so versatile. We always blitz leftover vegetables in the blender before adding them into the egg mix. They look so bright and delicious with beetroot! Charlotte loves that she can have a pink breakfast (we always make this when she has friends round).

Also, we make up a big batch of them at the start of the week and then just heat them up in a frying pan/skillet over the next few days.

---

serves 1

1 organic, free-range egg
1 tsp dried mixed herbs
1 small pre-cooked beetroot
pinch of salt and ground black pepper
1 tsp coconut oil
quarter of an avocado
half a lemon, cut in two
1 tsp fresh coriander/cilantro, chopped
salt and ground black pepper, to season
50 g/1¾ oz/⅓ cup smoked salmon
2 cherry tomatoes, chopped
handful of rocket/arugula

1. Put the egg, herbs, beetroot, salt and pepper into a blender. Mix well until everything is combined and the mixture is pink.

2. Heat a frying pan/skillet over a low heat and add the oil. Once the oil is melted, add the egg mixture and rotate the pan to let it all spread out thinly.

3. Leave to cook for approximately 3 minutes. Then flip the wrap on to the other side for another few minutes, until it is firm.

4. In a bowl, mash the avocado, squeeze in the juice from one of the two wedges of lemon and add some chopped coriander/cilantro (or any other herb you like). Season with salt and pepper.

5. Once the wrap is cooked, spread on the mashed avocado, add the smoked salmon and sprinkle the rocket/arugula and tomato on top. Squeeze over the juice from the remaining lemon wedge and season with more pepper. Roll it up firmly and enjoy.

Top Tip Keep them fresh in the fridge by placing a piece of parchment paper in-between each wrap.

THE EGG BOWL

This is the best possible start you can have to the day. If you want to be kind to yourself, it's the ideal place to begin. This is such a heart-warming comfort food and one of the few dishes where the taste matches its wonderful health benefits. It's one of those dishes that never fails you — and it can easily be served at any time of the day.

serves 2
for the lemon tahini dressing
3 tbsp tahini
Juice of 1 lemon
handful of cashews
handful of fresh parsley
salt and ground black pepper, to taste
120 ml/4 fl oz/½ cup water
drizzle of olive oil

for the bowl
3 tsp coconut oil
half a red onion, chopped
handful of pistachios, chopped
2 garlic cloves, crushed
150 g/5¼ oz/1 cup buckwheat groats
    (cooked in stock, according to instructions)
handful of fresh parsley, chopped, plus an
    extra sprig, to garnish
1 avocado, mashed, plus a few slices to
    garnish
juice of half a lemon
1 tsp chilli flakes
2 handfuls of fresh spinach
2 organic, free-range eggs
2 tbsp sauerkraut (optional)

1. Put all the dressing ingredients in a blender and whizz it up. Add more water until you get the perfect consistency. Season to taste.

2. Heat 1 teaspoon of the coconut oil in a frying pan/ skillet. Add the onion, pistachios and half the garlic and season. Leave to sauté until soft and cooked through. Add the cooked buckwheat and mix everything together. Season to taste and add in the parsley.

3. Mix the avocado with the lemon juice and chilli flakes. Season to taste.

4. In a frying pan/skillet, heat another 1 teaspoon of coconut oil and add the remaining garlic and then the spinach. Leave it to wilt.

5. Meanwhile, heat another frying pan/skillet, add the remaining 1 teaspoon of coconut oil and fry the eggs.

6. Serve the buckwheat equally into two bowls, followed by the smashed avocado, a big tablespoon of spinach and a tablespoon of sauerkraut (if using).

7. Place the fried eggs on the top of the bowls and drizzle with dressing and a sprig of parsley. Serve with the extra avocado slices.

AVOCADO, TOMATO AND CHILLI SALSA WITH QUINOA BREAD

I love smashed avo. I also love salsa. So I decided to mix them together! This salsa makes the perfect addition to... literally everything. Have it with eggs, smother it on toast, or add it to your chicken or fish dish. If you aren't a fan of spice, then lower the amount of chilli.

serves 4

3 avocados, peeled, stoned and diced
half a red chilli, deseeded and finely
    chopped
2-cm/¾-inch piece of fresh root ginger,
    finely grated
juice of 1 lime
½ tsp grated lime zest
1 spring onion/scallion, finely chopped
pinch of Himalayan pink salt
small handful of fresh mint, chopped
small handful of fresh coriander/cilantro,
    chopped
150 g/5¼ oz/¾ cup cherry tomatoes,
    quartered

for the bread

85 g/3 oz/½ cup uncooked quinoa, cooked
    with a pinch of salt, drained and cooled
85 g/3 oz/½ cup linseeds/flaxseeds
140 g/5 oz/1 cup sunflower seeds, soaked
    for about 1 hour
130 g/4½ oz/1 cup pumpkin seeds
2 tbsp chia seeds
4 tbsp psyllium husks
1 tsp Himalayan pink salt
3 tbsp coconut oil, melted
350 ml/12 fl oz/1½ cups lukewarm water
1 tbsp maple syrup or honey

1. Start by making the bread. In a bowl, combine the quinoa along with the dry ingredients.

2. In a separate bowl, mix the coconut oil with the water and maple syrup or honey.

3. Combine the wet ingredients with the dry and stir until the mixture starts to thicken.

4. Line a 450-g/1-lb loaf tin with parchment paper, pour in the mixture and allow to set for at least an hour or overnight.

5. Preheat the oven to 180°C/350°F/gas mark 4.

6. Bake in the preheated oven for 45 minutes or until browned and pulling away from the parchment paper. Remove from the oven, allow to cool slightly and remove from the tin and parchment paper, then return to the oven for up to 15 minutes to brown the outside.

7. To make the avocado salsa, simply mash the avocados in a mixing bowl. Add in all of the remaining ingredients and mix really well. Season to taste.

8. Slice the bread and toast it under the grill/broiler. Spread on the salsa and enjoy. If you want to get all extravagant, then serve with a poached egg or two.

HEALTHY BREAKFAST HASH

This is a really filling breakfast that is a great vehicle for any leftover cooked or raw vegetables. If using potatoes, cook them from room temperature and give them a good five-minute head start on your other ingredients in the pan, as they take the longest to cook. Put a lid on the pan while cooking the potatoes to help speed things up. At the end, when cracking in the eggs, make sure the pan is off the heat so the bottom of the eggs don't burn; eggs are always best cooked low and slow.

serves 2

1 potato, diced into small cubes
1 sweet potato, diced into small cubes
1 tbsp coconut oil
1 red pepper, finely diced
2 spring onions/scallions, chopped
handful of spinach or kale, chopped
¼ tsp salt
¼ tsp ground black pepper
2 organic, free-range eggs
pinch of chilli flakes (optional)
fresh coriander/cilantro or parsley, to serve

1. Put the potatoes into a saucepan filled with boiling water and leave to cook for approximately 10 minutes, until cooked through, then drain.

2. Heat the oil in a medium-sized frying pan/skillet.

3. Throw the potatoes in and put the lid on. Every few minutes, give the potatoes a toss to ensure they are browning but not burning; having the lid on cooks them faster because they are searing and steaming at the same time.

4. After about 5 minutes of cooking time, turn down the heat and throw in the finely diced pepper, spinach and spring onions/scallions.

5. Add the salt and ground black pepper and cook for another minute.

6. Take the pan off the heat, make room in the pan and crack in the eggs. Season the eggs with a pinch of chilli flakes and salt and pepper, if you like.

7. Put the pan back over a medium to low heat and put the lid on.

8. Cook the eggs for about 2 minutes, or more if you like them well done.

9. Serve up the hash onto plates and put the eggs on top. Sprinkle with your freshly chopped herb of choice and enjoy a satisfying breakfast.

BRUNCHY BAKED EGGS

This is the perfect dish for a weekend brunch — it tastes delicious and looks impressive. Bear in mind that it's near impossible to get all the eggs baked to the same level — the ones in the middle will be runny and the ones at the edge crispy.

serves 4

280 g/10 oz/4 packed cups fresh spinach
1 tbsp olive oil or butter
1 small white onion, finely diced
2 garlic cloves, crushed
140 g/5 oz/2 cups mushrooms, chopped
3 tbsp single/light cream
pinch of freshly grated nutmeg (a little goes a long way)
¼ tsp salt
¼ tsp ground black pepper
4 large, organic, free-range eggs
1 tbsp grated Parmesan or a sprinkling of feta (optional)

1. Preheat the oven to 180°C/350°F/gas mark 4.

2. First, cook the spinach in a small pot of boiling water until just wilted. This should only take 2 minutes.

3. Drain the spinach, and once cool, squeeze the liquid out of it with your hands and roughly chop it up.

4. Heat the oil or butter over a medium heat in an ovenproof frying pan/skillet and sauté the onion for 3 minutes, until softened.

5. Add the garlic and cook for another minute.

6. Add the mushrooms and stir, allowing the mix to cook for another 3 minutes.

7. Add in your drained, chopped spinach, the cream, nutmeg, salt and pepper. Stir everything together and let the flavours distribute evenly while bringing to a simmer for 1–2 minutes.

8. Take the pan off the heat and make 4 indentations in the mixture with the back of a big spoon.

9. Crack an egg into each dent, sprinkle lightly with salt and pepper and put the pan in your oven. Leave it to cook for about 6 minutes and check it.

10. You want the whites to have set but the yolks to be runny. If the egg whites still look raw, give it another 2 minutes in the oven.

11. Take the dish out and sprinkle the cheese on top, if desired. Serve up immediately with buttered slices of your favourite toast, or enjoy on its own!

BUCKWHEAT, EGG, CARROT AND MUSHROOM CRÊPES

Breakfast crêpe recipes are generally laden with sugary sweet fillings; this savoury crêpe is something I discovered in Australia and it's perfect for brunch or even lunch. I love the addition of the crunchy sweet carrots and thyme in this dish. Buckwheat crêpes are beautifully light so it is important to keep the batter in the fridge, because it keeps them fluffy and delicious.

serves 4

330 g/11½ oz/2¾ cups buckwheat flour
2 tsp Himalayan pink salt
750 ml/1¼ pints/3 cups filtered water
5 organic, free-range eggs
3 carrots
5 large portobello mushrooms
2 tbsp coconut oil
1 tbsp fresh thyme leaves
280 g/10 oz/4 packed cups fresh spinach
salt and ground black pepper, to season
1 tsp black sesame seeds, to garnish

1. Combine the flour and salt and gradually add the water, a little at a time, stirring after each addition. Add one egg and incorporate into the mixture. Put the batter in the fridge for 1–2 hours, because this will make the crêpes nice and fluffy.

2. While the batter is in the fridge, coarsely grate the carrot and finely slice the mushrooms. Heat 1 tablespoon of the coconut oil in a frying pan/skillet and lightly fry the mushrooms with the fresh thyme. After 2 minutes, stir in the spinach and cook until the spinach is wilted. This should take 5 minutes. Remove from the heat and set aside.

3. Heat the remaining coconut oil in a non-stick frying pan/skillet and ladle in the crêpe mixture, swirling it around the pan to create a nice thin layer. Fry until the edges start to crisp and then flip over and cook on the other side. Repeat this process for all the crêpes and set aside. Meanwhile, fry the remaining eggs in a separate pan.

4. Place a crêpe on a plate and sprinkle a quarter of the grated carrot, mushroom and spinach mixture down the middle. Season, then top with a fried egg and fold over. Garnish with black sesame seeds.

Top Tip This dish is delicious with a spoonful of Homemade Harissa (see page 185).

LUNCH

BOWLS

Bowls are the foodie way forward. The amazing thing about them is that you can mix and match each part to tailor-make your very own nutrient-rich lunch. You can make a large amount of each component and just spoon it into a container each day, or you can make the bowls look beautiful and invite a load of friends round to enjoy them together. Choose your base, add the protein, veggies and a spoon of dip on top. Each bowl serves 4.

IMMUNE BOWL

for the base (brown rice)

160 g/5⅔ oz/¾ cup brown rice

500 ml/17 fl oz/2 cups bone broth (see Miracle Bone Broth recipe on page 159), or if you don't have bone broth, use stock instead

500 ml/17 fl oz/2 cups water

salt and ground black pepper, to season

1 tbsp olive oil

1 onion, chopped

1 garlic clove, crushed

1. Wash the brown rice in a sieve/strainer before placing it in a large saucepan. Add the broth and water, and place over a high heat to bring to the boil. Once it's boiling, lower the heat. Season with salt and pepper. Leave to cook for 15–20 minutes, until the rice is cooked through.

2. In a frying pan/skillet, add the olive oil and place over a low heat. Add the onion and garlic and leave to sauté for approximately 5 minutes, until the onion has softened.

3. Pour the onion and garlic into the saucepan and mix through.

for the protein (turkey meatballs)

500 g/1 lb 2 oz/2¼ cups minced/ground turkey

2 carrots, grated

1 courgette/zucchini, grated

2 tbsp tomato purée/paste

2 tbsp mixed Italian seasoning

1 onion

salt and ground black pepper, to season

1 organic, free-range egg

1 tbsp coconut oil

1. Place the minced/ground turkey in a mixing bowl. Stir in the carrots, courgette/zucchini, tomato purée/paste, Italian seasoning and the onion. Season with salt and pepper and mix. Stir in the egg.

2. Wet your hands and roll a tablespoon of the mixture into a ball and place on a baking tray. Continue to do this until all the mixture is used up — it should be enough for 12 balls.

3. Heat a large frying pan/skillet over a medium heat and add the oil. Once it is melted, cook the meatballs for 5–6 minutes, or until cooked through and nicely browned on the outside. You'll probably have to repeat the process for a second batch, unless you have a large frying pan.

for the veggies (charred broccoli and chilli)

2 heads of broccoli (about 500 g/1 lb 2 oz),
     cut into florets
115 ml/4 fl oz/½ cup olive oil
coarse sea salt and freshly ground black
     pepper
4 garlic cloves, thinly sliced
1 red chilli, deseeded and thinly sliced
50 g/1¾ oz/⅔ cup flaked/slivered almonds,
     toasted

1. Fill a large saucepan with water and bring to the boil. Throw in the broccoli and blanch for 2 minutes. Drain the broccoli and transfer it to a bowl full of ice-cold water. Drain and use paper towels to dry completely. In a mixing bowl, toss the broccoli with 3 tablespoons of the oil and a generous pinch of salt and pepper.

2. Place a griddle/grill pan over a high heat until it is extremely hot (approximately 3 minutes). Grill the broccoli in several batches, turning them around as they grill so they get char marks all over. Transfer to a heatproof bowl and continue with another batch

3. While grilling the broccoli, place the remaining oil in a small saucepan with the garlic and chilli. Cook them over a medium heat until the garlic just begins to turn golden brown. Be careful not to let the garlic and chilli burn. Pour the oil mixture over the hot broccoli and mix together well. Taste and adjust the seasoning.

4. Garnish the broccoli with almonds before serving.

for the dip (ratatouille)

1 tbsp rapeseed oil
1 onion, chopped
2 garlic cloves, crushed
salt and ground black pepper, to season
2 x 400-g/14-oz cans organic chopped
     tomatoes
1 tbsp dried oregano
1 tbsp red wine vinegar
1 tbsp tomato purée/paste
2 peppers, deseeded and chopped

1. Heat the oil in a large saucepan. Add the onion and garlic and leave to sauté over a low heat for 5 minutes, until the onion softens. Season with salt and pepper.

2. Pour in the tomatoes, oregano, vinegar, purée/paste and peppers and stir well. Cook over a low heat for 15–20 minutes.

OMEGA-3 BOWL

for the base (kelp noodles)
340 g/12 oz/3 cups kelp noodles
2 tbsp tamari
4 tbsp sesame oil
60 g/2 oz/½ cup cashews, toasted and
   chopped

1. Rinse the kelp noodles in warm water for about 10 minutes. This will soften and separate them. Drain the noodles and, using kitchen scissors, cut them into small pieces.

2. Mix the kelp noodles with the tamari and sesame oil. Stir in the toasted cashews.

---

for the protein (miso-glazed salmon)
1 tbsp miso paste
2-cm/¾-inch piece of fresh root ginger,
   grated
4 tbsp coconut milk
2 tbsp tamari
3 spring onions/scallions, finely chopped
juice of 1 lime
4 organic salmon fillets (approximately
   250 g/9 oz)

1. Preheat the oven to 180°C/350°F/gas mark 4.

2. Whisk the miso paste, ginger, coconut milk, tamari, spring onions/scallions and lime together to make the marinade and season to taste.

3. Place the salmon fillets in a deep ovenproof dish and pour the marinade into the dish. Cover with foil. Leave to marinate for a minimum of 2 hours (or overnight).

4. Place in the oven for 12–15 minutes, until cooked. Once cool, slice into flakes.

---

for the veggies (pak choi/bok choy and chilli)
1 tbsp sesame oil
1 tbsp coconut oil
1 large garlic clove, crushed
half a red chilli, deseeded and finely
   chopped
1 pak choi/bok choy
1 tbsp tamari

1. Place a lidded wok over a medium heat and add the oils. Once melted, add the garlic and chilli and lower the heat. Leave to sauté for 2–3 minutes.

2. Add the pak choi/bok choy and toss until coated with the garlic and chilli mixture. Cover with the lid and leave to cook for 5 minutes.

3. Take the wok off the heat. Pour over the tamari and toss well.

for the dip (edamame bean and ginger dip)
230 g/8 oz/1½ cups frozen shelled
    edamame beans
60 ml/2 fl oz/¼ cup water
2 tbsp tamari
2 tsp fresh root ginger, minced
1 tbsp rice vinegar
1 tbsp tahini
1 garlic clove, chopped
pinch of salt

1. Cook the edamame beans as instructed on
   the packet.

2. Add all the ingredients into a blender and blitz
   until smooth.

3. Season to taste.

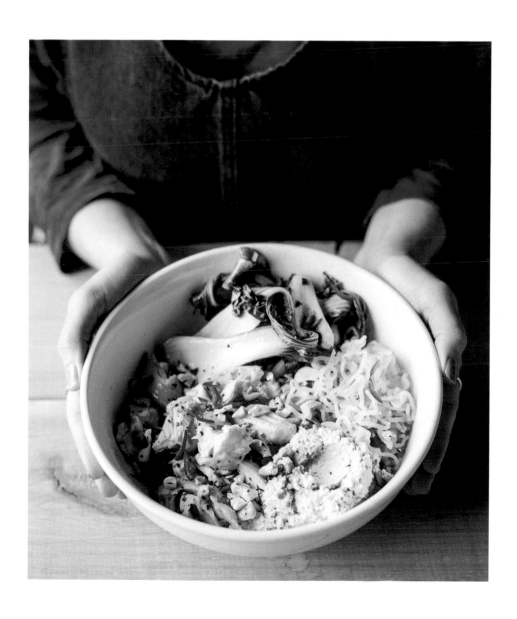

HAPPY BOWL

for the base (cauliflower rice)
2 cauliflowers, florets only
1 tsp coconut oil
1 onion, finely chopped
2 garlic cloves, crushed
salt and ground black pepper, to season

1. To make the cauliflower rice, pulse the cauliflower in the bowl of a food processor until it resembles rice (about 2–3 minutes); set aside.

2. Heat a large frying pan/skillet over a low heat and add the oil. Add the onion and garlic and leave to sauté for 5 minutes, until the onion is soft.

3. Mix in the cauliflower rice.

4. Season to taste.

for the protein (harissa chicken)
4 organic chicken breasts (approximately
    150 g/5¼ oz each)
4 tbsp Homemade Harissa (see page 185),
    or opt for a good-quality shop-bought one
    with no added sugar
1 tbsp coconut oil
2 red onions, quartered

1. Coat the chicken with harissa.

2. Heat a large griddle/grill pan over a medium heat. Once hot, add the coconut oil. When it has melted, add the chicken and cook on each side for 3–4 minutes, until lightly charred and cooked through.

3. Add the onions after the chicken has been cooking for 4 minutes and leave to sauté for 5 minutes until the onion is soft. Remove from the heat.

**for the veggies (wilted spinach, garlic and
    pine nuts)**
800 g/1¾ lb/11 packed cups fresh spinach
3 tbsp rapeseed oil
2 garlic cloves, finely chopped
3 tbsp pine nuts

1. Wash the spinach and place into a large saucepan. Pour over a little boiling water and cover for 2–3 minutes while the spinach wilts.

2. Drain the spinach in a colander.

3. In a frying pan/skillet, heat the oil and add the garlic and pine nuts. Fry until golden (approximately 3 minutes).

4. Stir in the spinach and season to taste.

for the dip (adzuki bean mash):
1 tsp coconut oil
1 onion, finely chopped
1 garlic clove, crushed
2 tsp ground cumin
1 tsp ground coriander
salt and ground black pepper, to season
1 x 400-g/14-oz can organic adzuki beans,
  drained
80 ml/2¾ fl oz/⅓ cup water

1. Heat a frying pan/skillet and add the oil. Once melted, add the onion and garlic and sauté for 5 minutes, until the onion has softened.

2. Add the cumin and coriander and mix well. Season with salt and pepper.

3. Pour the drained beans and the water into a blender. Pour in the onion and garlic mixture.

4. Blend until all the ingredients are well combined.

MIDDLE EASTERN BOWL

for the base (quinoa)
200 g/7 oz/1 cup uncooked quinoa
2 tsp ground turmeric
juice of 1 lemon
2 tbsp tamari
20 g/¾ oz/⅓ cup fresh parsley, finely chopped
20 g/¾ oz/⅓ cup fresh coriander/cilantro, finely
   chopped
2 spring onions/scallions, finely chopped

1. Rinse the quinoa in water to remove its bitter flavour. Tip into a large saucepan and add salted water to a volume that is approximately double that of the quinoa. Add the turmeric, lemon juice and tamari. Place on the boil for 15 minutes, until the quinoa is cooked but still retains a slight bite.

2. Fluff it up with a fork and then mix in the parsley, coriander/cilantro and spring onions/scallions. Season to taste.

for the protein (beetroot falafel)
150 g/5¼ oz/¾ cup uncooked chickpeas
1 garlic clove, crushed
1 tsp paprika
150 g/5¼ oz/¾ cup cooked beetroot,
   chopped
1 lemon, zest only
1 tbsp fresh coriander/cilantro, finely
   chopped
1 tbsp buckwheat flour
½ tsp bicarbonate of soda/baking soda

1. Soak the chickpeas in water and a pinch of salt overnight. In the morning, drain and dry thoroughly.

2. Preheat the oven to 180°C/350°F/gas mark 4 and line a baking tray with parchment paper.

3. Heat the oil in a frying pan/skillet and add the garlic and paprika. Leave to sauté for 2–3 minutes.

4. Pour the chickpeas, beetroot, garlic mixture, lemon and coriander/cilantro into a food processor and whizz it up. Add the flour and bicarbonate of soda/baking soda and blend again.

5. Using damp hands, roll the mixture into even-sized balls and place on the baking tray. Brush lightly with oil and bake for 20–25 minutes, until crisp and warm.

for the veggies (Israeli salad)
1 cucumber, diced
4 plum tomatoes, deseeded and finely
   chopped
1 red pepper, finely chopped
40 g/1½ oz/⅔ cup fresh parsley, chopped
40 g/1½ oz/⅔ cup fresh mint, chopped
juice of 1 lemon
50 ml/2 fl oz/¼ cup olive oil
salt and ground black pepper, to season

1. In a bowl, mix the cucumber, tomatoes, pepper, parsley and mint.

2. Add the lemon juice and oil and mix well. Season to taste.

for the dip (butternut squash hummus)
200 g/7 oz/1½ cups butternut/winter
  squash, peeled and chopped into cubes
2 garlic cloves, peeled
1 tbsp coconut oil, melted
juice of 1 lemon
1 x 400-g/14-oz can chickpeas, drained and
  rinsed
2 tbsp tahini
4 tbsp olive oil
2 tbsp fresh coriander/cilantro, chopped
salt and ground black pepper, to season

1. Preheat the oven to 180°C/350°F/gas mark 4 and line
   a baking tray with parchment paper.

2. Place the squash and garlic cloves on the tray and
   drizzle with coconut oil. Place in the preheated oven
   for 20 minutes, until cooked through. Leave to cool.

3. Put the squash into a food processor. Add all the
   other ingredients apart from one of the garlic cloves
   and mix until well combined. Season to taste.

FISH FINGER SANDWICH

This is the Bodyism take on a fish-finger sandwich for when you want some pure comfort food — your body will thank you for it.

serves 2
280 g/10 oz/4 packed cups fresh spinach
4 slices organic sourdough bread
2 handfuls of sliced iceberg lettuce
sweet potato fries, to serve
lemon wedges, to serve

for the tartare sauce
3 tbsp organic Greek yoghurt
½ tsp horseradish
1 heaped tbsp chopped fresh chives
salt and ground black pepper, to season

for the smashed avocado
1 avocado
juice of half a lemon
pinch of chilli flakes
salt and ground black pepper, to season

for the fish fingers
100 g/3½ oz/¾ cup buckwheat flour
100 g/3½ oz/¾ cup brown rice flour
100 g/3½ oz/1 cup ground almonds
1 tsp garlic powder
1 tsp dried parsley
1 lemon, zest only
salt and ground black pepper, to season
3 organic, free-range eggs
200 g/7 oz organic (or locally sourced), skinless haddock loin (or any other line-caught white fish)
2 tsp rapeseed oil or olive oil

1. Heat the grill/broiler to medium temperature.

2. Mix the tartare sauce ingredients together and leave in the fridge while you make everything else.

3. Make the smashed avocado by mashing the avocado add adding the lemon juice, chilli flakes and salt and pepper. Mix well.

4. For the fish fingers, mix the buckwheat flour, rice flour, almonds, garlic powder, parsley, lemon zest, salt and pepper in a bowl and mix well.

5. In a separate bowl, crack the eggs and whisk.

6. Slice the haddock into 4 chunky fingers.

7. Dip one piece of fish at a time into the egg and then the flour mix. To make them extra crunchy, repeat this step.

8. Put a frying pan/skillet over a medium heat and add a splash of oil. When the pan is hot, add the fingers (you might need to do this in batches) and fry for approximately 3 minutes each side, or until they are cooked through, golden and crispy. Remove to a double layer of paper towels to drain while you fry the next batch (add more oil if needed).

9. Grill/broil the bread while the fish is cooking.

10. Spread the smashed avocado on 2 slices of the toasted bread. Put a handful of iceberg lettuce on top of each, followed by two fish fingers. Finish each sandwich with the remaining toast, spread with the tartare sauce. Serve on a plate with sweet potato fries and lemon wedges.

MISO PRAWN AND AUBERGINE SALAD

I love this Asian-inspired salad; it's the perfect combination of sweet (from the coconut) and salt (from the tamari). Most dressings are packed with sugar, so make sure you read the bottle if you opt for a shop-bought one. Aubergines/eggplants are such great additions to salads because they are quite filling, they absorb the dressing really well and are really easy to cook. If you don't want prawns/shrimp, then add any other protein you fancy — chicken, salmon, turkey or some chickpeas.

serves 4

400 g/14 oz buckwheat soba noodles
1 tbsp coconut oil
2 aubergines/eggplants, diced
half a red chilli, deseeded and finely chopped
12 large raw tiger prawns/shrimp
2 tbsp coconut milk
100 g/3½ oz/⅓ cup brown miso paste
2 tbsp sesame oil
3 tbsp tamari
4-cm/1½-inch piece of fresh root ginger, grated
1 tbsp rice wine vinegar
4 spring onions/scallions, finely chopped
50 g/1¾ oz/⅔ cup coconut flakes, toasted
fresh coriander/cilantro leaves, to serve

1. Bring a pan of water to the boil and cook the noodles following the packet instructions.

2. Heat the coconut oil in a large frying pan/skillet until melted. Cook the aubergines/eggplant and chilli over a medium heat for 8–10 minutes, until softened.

3. In the last few minutes of cooking the aubergine/eggplant, throw in the prawns/shrimp and leave them to turn opaque — it should take about 3 minutes.

4. Mix together the coconut milk, miso, sesame oil, tamari, ginger and vinegar.

5. Drain the noodles and add to the pan of prawns/shrimp and aubergines/eggplants. Pour over the dressing and serve with a scattering of spring onions/scallions, toasted coconut and coriander/cilantro leaves.

CHICKPEA DOSA WRAP

I love a wrap and I throw anything I can find into it! This chickpea wrap is one of my absolute favourites because it is so easy to make. Often, I make them in bulk and then just grab one from the fridge when I'm in a rush. Experiment with adding different dried spices and herbs into the batter.

serves 4

250 g/8¾ oz/2 cups chickpea/gram flour
salt and ground black pepper, to season
400 ml/14 fl oz/1⅔ cups water
1 tbsp coconut oil
1 garlic clove, crushed
1 shallot, finely chopped
half a red pepper, finely chopped
1 tbsp rapeseed oil

for the filling

2 tbsp Butternut Squash Hummus (see page 129)
half an avocado, sliced
1 plum tomato, sliced
slices of Harissa Chicken (see page 126), or any other fillings you fancy

1. Put the flour in a mixing bowl and season with salt and pepper. Make a well in the centre of the flour and pour in the water slowly, while whisking, until well combined. Set aside for at least half an hour.

2. Heat a 20-cm/8-inch frying pan/skillet and add the coconut oil. Add the garlic, shallot and red pepper. Sauté over a low heat for 5 minutes, until the shallot has softened. Take off the heat and leave to cool.

3. Pour the shallot, garlic and red pepper into the flour mixture and stir well.

4. Heat a small frying pan/skillet and add the rapeseed oil. Once the pan is very hot and the oil has spread across the pan, pour in a small ladle of the batter. Spread the mixture across the base of the pan and leave to cook for approximately 3 minutes. Using a spatula, flip the dosa over and leave to cook on the other side. Remove from the pan and repeat until all the batter is used up.

5. Spread the hummus on each wrap and pile up with fillings. Wrap up and enjoy!

KABBOULEH

This is a delicious lunch-box treat or the perfect accompaniment to any protein. Feel free to mix up your grains and use what you have to hand — simply sauté any leftover grains in a little olive oil rather than cooking them fresh. If you're gluten-intolerant, avoid couscous and bulgur wheat, and use quinoa or brown rice instead. Use this salad as a vehicle for leftover vegetables — the choice is yours!

serves 4

3 tbsp extra virgin olive oil
¼ tsp ground cumin
½ tsp sumac
juice of 1 lemon
¼ tsp salt
¼ tsp ground black pepper
3 handfuls of kale (stalks discarded), finely chopped
half a small cucumber, seeds scooped out, finely chopped
1 spring onion/scallion, finely chopped
8 small tomatoes, chopped into quarters
handful of fresh parsley, finely chopped
100 g/3½ oz/½ cup cooked and cooled quinoa, brown rice or bulgur wheat (or any leftover cooked grains you have)

1. First, make the dressing; it will only taste better the longer it sits. Whisk together the olive oil, cumin, sumac, lemon juice, salt and pepper and set aside.

2. Put the kale, cucumber, spring onion/scallion and tomatoes into a serving bowl and stir in the parsley.

3. Pour over half the dressing and mix it through; this step will tenderize the kale and distribute great flavour through the salad.

4. Add in your cooled grains and the rest of your dressing, stirring everything together. It's important to make sure the grains have cooled down completely before adding them, so they don't wilt the salad — you want fresh, crisp bites, not soggy ones.

5. Taste the salad for seasoning and add more salt or another squeeze of lemon if needed. Make it your own and add as much or as little of the seasonings as you like! Tuck in and enjoy every bite.

Top Tip If you like heat, feel free to add in a little fresh or dried chilli, or some finely chopped garlic.

BODYISM FRITTATA

This is such a delicious way to use up any leftover vegetables in the fridge. Use this recipe as your guide and feel free to swap any vegetables or herbs with what you have available.

serves 4

1 tbsp coconut oil
2 garlic cloves, crushed
3 courgettes/zucchini, sliced into discs
1 leek, sliced
4 mushrooms, sliced
8 organic, free-range eggs
salt and ground black pepper, to season
1 tbsp dried mixed herbs
handful of vegetables (leftover roasted
    squash, parsnips, red pepper or peas from
    the freezer)
handful of organic Cheddar, grated (optional)

1. Heat the grill/broiler to high.

2. Heat a large ovenproof frying pan/skillet on the hob/stovetop and add the coconut oil. Once melted, add the garlic, courgettes/zucchini, leek and mushrooms. Leave to sauté for 5–8 minutes, until the leek and courgettes/zucchini are soft. Leave to cool.

3. Beat the eggs in a bowl and season well. Add the mixed herbs and all the vegetables.

4. Pour the egg mixture into the frying pan/skillet with the vegetables and cook over a low heat for 8–10 minutes.

5. If you are adding cheese, sprinkle on top and place in the grill/broiler for 3–5 minutes, until set.

6. Cut into thick wedges and serve. This also makes a delicious breakfast — so keep the leftovers and enjoy the next day.

ALKALIZING SUPERGREEN SOUP

This soup is filled with alkalizing greens and nourishing broth. It is one of those dishes that will make you feel a little bit smug because it is just so ridiculously good for you. The key with soups and stews is to build the flavour by seasoning as you go and to follow the initial steps properly. In this case, make sure you have sautéed the onions until translucent and given the garlic a minute or two to cook before adding the parsnip and broth. These initial steps will really bring a sweetness and depth of flavour to the soup. If you want a thicker soup, feel free to add extra parsnip.

This soup will keep in your fridge for up to three days. I like to eat half and freeze the rest for a rainy day.

serves 4, with leftovers

1 tbsp olive oil
1 large white onion, chopped
2 large garlic cloves, crushed
½ tsp salt
½ tsp freshly ground pepper
1 parsnip, peeled and diced into small cubes
1 l/1¾ pints/4 cups chicken stock or vegetable stock (top up with hot water, if desired)
2 large handfuls of kale (stalks discarded)
4 large handfuls of fresh spinach
1 large handful of cavolo nero (stalks discarded)

1. Heat the olive oil in a large pot over a medium heat. Sauté the onion until translucent, for about 2 minutes.

2. Add the garlic and half the salt and pepper and allow to cook for about 2 minutes. You don't want to add the stock while the garlic is raw.

3. Add in your diced parsnip and stir. Pour in 1 litre of whatever stock you have chosen (I prefer chicken stock) and top up with hot water, if desired.

4. Add the kale, spinach and cavolo nero. Turn up the heat and allow the soup to come to a boil, then turn down to a low simmer.

5. Add the remaining salt and pepper and stir in. Let the soup simmer and the flavours develop for about 20 minutes.

6. Blend to a smooth consistency using a food processor or hand-held blender (be careful, please!) and simmer over a low heat for another 30 minutes.

7. Taste and add more salt or pepper, or perhaps a dash of cream for richness, if desired.

8. Make the soup your own and enjoy!

TURMERIC, SWEET POTATO, GINGER AND COCONUT SOUP

This is such a bright and beautiful soup. It's filled with nourishing ingredients to zap away those change-of-weather colds. I like making a big batch and freezing it for a simple supper. It's the perfect autumnal soup.

serves 5

1 tbsp coconut oil
2 red onions, diced
1 head of celery, diced
thumb of fresh root ginger, grated
3 medium-sized sweet potatoes, peeled and
    cut into chunks
2 tsp ground turmeric
1 x 400-ml/14-fl oz can organic coconut milk
juice of 1 lime
fresh coriander/cilantro, to serve

1. Heat the coconut oil in a large, heavy-based saucepan until melted. Add the red onions and the celery and sauté for 5 minutes.

2. Add the grated ginger and sweet potato and simmer for a further 5 minutes. Cover with boiling water, so the pan is about two-thirds full.

3. Add the turmeric and simmer for 15 minutes, until the sweet potato is soft.

4. Turn off the heat, add the coconut milk and blend with a hand-held blender or food processor.

5. Pour back into the saucepan and simmer, being careful not to bring to the boil.

6. Add the lime juice and season to taste. Pour into bowls and garnish with coriander/cilantro.

Top Tip The sweet potato can be substituted with squash to make a delicious bright and light soup.

DINNER

COURGETTE LASAGNE

This lasagne is a much healthier version than the traditional recipe, but that doesn't take away from its taste. The meat sauce is packed with flavour, and I like to leave it cooking away for hours, just to make it all the more intense. If you want, you can swap the courgette/zucchini with layers of thinly sliced squash or sweet potato, but I do like the courgette/zucchini best.

serves 4

1 tbsp coconut oil
1 onion, chopped
2 garlic cloves, finely chopped
1 tsp ground nutmeg
1 tsp ground cinnamon
1 tbsp dried oregano
handful of fresh basil, finely chopped
2 tbsp tomato purée/paste
1 tsp Worcestershire sauce
500 g/1 lb 2 oz lean organic minced/ground
   lamb
1 x 400-g/14-oz can chopped tomatoes
1 tbsp red wine vinegar
4 courgettes/zucchini, sliced into ribbons
   with a peeler
75 g/2⅔ oz/1 cup mushrooms, sliced
Parmesan, grated

1. Preheat the oven to 200°C/400°F/gas mark 6.

2. Heat the oil in a large frying pan/skillet over a medium heat and sauté the onion and garlic for approximately 5 minutes, until softened.

3. Add the nutmeg, cinnamon, oregano, basil, tomato purée/paste and Worcestershire sauce and mix well. Add the lamb and cook for 10 minutes, until brown.

4. Stir in the tomatoes and vinegar and simmer for 15–20 minutes.

5. In a large baking dish, spoon a layer of the mixture, topped with a layer of courgette/zucchini ribbons and then a layer of mushrooms. Repeat, finishing with a layer of courgette/zucchini ribbons.

6. Sprinkle the Parmesan over the top and bake for 15–20 minutes.

7. Serve with a fresh green salad.

ULTIMATE FISH PIE

Fish pie reminds me of after-school dinners. Full of flavour, protein and vegetables, it's one of those home comforts, and this version is wonderful for you, too.

    This is a dish that you can really play with and adapt to your own tastes. Use any firm white fish, from cod to pollock. Vary up the mash — try creamy potatoes, swede/rutabaga or even cauliflower — it's entirely up to you. Get your mash started first, so the celeriac can boil while you're preparing the pie.

serves 4

½ tsp butter
½ tsp olive oil
1 white onion, chopped
2 large garlic cloves, minced
2 carrots, peeled and chopped
1 leek, white part only, chopped
½ tsp salt
½ tsp ground black pepper
700 ml/1¼ pints/3 cups whole milk
1 bay leaf
1 tbsp arrowroot powder
400 g/14 oz cod, chopped into bite-sized
    chunks
200 g/7 oz smoked haddock, chopped into
    bite-sized chunks
175 g/6 oz prawns/shrimp
large handful of fresh parsley, including
    stalks, chopped

for the mash

2 small celeriac, peeled and cut into chunks
pinch of salt
¼ tsp ground black pepper
½ tbsp butter

1. Preheat the oven to 180°C/350°F/gas mark 4.

2. To make the mash, add the celeriac and salt to a pot of water and bring to the boil. Turn the heat down and simmer gently for 20 minutes. Drain and mash the celeriac, adding the pepper and butter. Set aside.

3. Put the butter and olive oil together in a large frying pan/skillet and melt over a medium heat. Add the onion and sauté for 3 minutes, until softened.

4. Add the garlic and sauté for another 1–2 minutes, until you can smell its garlicky aroma. Add the carrots and leek and half the salt and pepper, and stir everything together.

5. Turn the heat down and pour in the milk, also adding the bay leaf. After it has heated for 1–2 minutes, scoop a ladleful of the milk mixture into a cup and whisk in the arrowroot. This will thicken the sauce.

6. Add the whisked milk and arrowroot back into the pan and stir. Add the fish and prawns/shrimp. The fish will poach in the milk and impart a lovely smoky flavour into the dish.

7. Add another pinch of salt and pepper to the liquid and throw in all the parsley. Allow this mix to simmer for about 6 minutes, until the fish is cooked.

8. Transfer the mixture to a baking dish. Top with the mash and place in the preheated oven. Bake for 25 minutes until bubbling at the edges.

DUKKAH-CRUSTED SALMON WITH ASIAN BRUSSELS SPROUT SALAD

This is another easy dinner recipe, which you can get ready in less than 30 minutes. Dukkah is such an easy rub to store and use when you need to make something delicious quickly. I even like it sprinkled over eggs or vegetables. Brussels sprouts were ruined when some stupid person told us to boil them; please try roasting them before you say you 'hate' sprouts.

serves 4

2 tbsp tamari
1 tsp garlic powder
400 g/14 oz/4 cups Brussels sprouts, halved
2 tbsp sesame oil
2 garlic cloves, thinly sliced
½ red chilli, deseeded and finely chopped
1 small red onion, chopped
2 pak choi/bok choy
50 g/1¾ oz/½ cup flaked/slivered almonds, toasted
1 tsp coconut oil
4 x 150 g/5¼ oz organic salmon fillets
fresh coriander/cilantro leaves, to serve

for the dukkah

3 tbsp coriander seeds
2 tbsp cumin seeds
40 g/1½ oz/¼ cup sesame seeds
300 g/10½ oz/3 cups pistachios, toasted
salt and ground black pepper, to season

1. Preheat the oven to 180°C/350°F/gas mark 4.

2. To make the dukkah, dry fry the seeds in a small frying pan/skillet over a low heat for 2 minutes (until fragrant and toasted). Leave to cool, then place them in a food processor with the pistachios. Blend until the mixture is crumb-like. Season to taste and leave to one side.

3. Meanwhile, melt the coconut oil and mix with the tamari and garlic powder. Place the Brussels sprouts in a baking tray and drizzle over the oil mixture. Cook in the preheated oven for 30 minutes, until nicely roasted. Once cooked, leave to cool.

4. Heat a lidded wok over a medium–high heat, add the sesame oil and, once piping hot, add the garlic, chilli and red onion. Sauté for 5 minutes, until the onion is soft. Add the pak choi/bok choy and cover the wok for 2 minutes. Take off the heat. Add the Brussels sprouts and almonds. Mix well.

5. Heat the coconut oil in a large frying pan/skillet. Roll the salmon in the dukkah mixture. Fry the salmon over a low heat for 3 minutes each side, or until cooked to your liking (I like it slightly raw in the middle).

6. Serve with the Brussels sprout salad and a sprinkling of fresh coriander/cilantro.

TURMERIC DHAL

If a cold is brewing, or it's one of those cold wintery nights and all you want to do is put your feet up on the sofa and not spend your evening preparing dinner, this is the answer. This Turmeric Dhal can sit on the hob/stovetop simmering away for hours (getting tastier and tastier). I could eat this for breakfast, lunch and dinner. It's great for breakfast, with a fried egg on the top.

serves 4

400 g/14 oz/2 cups red lentils
1 tbsp coconut oil
4 onions, sliced
8 garlic cloves, crushed
80 g/2¾ oz fresh, unpeeled ginger root, grated
half a red chilli, deseeded and finely chopped
1 tbsp ground coriander
1 tbsp ground cumin
1 tbsp ground turmeric
1 tsp garam masala
1 tsp ground cinnamon
2 leeks, sliced into discs
2 carrots, finely diced
2 celery sticks, finely diced
1 l/1¾ pints/4 cups bone broth (see Miracle Bone Broth on page 159) or vegetable stock
3 large handfuls of fresh coriander/cilantro, stalks finely chopped and leaves roughly chopped, plus extra to serve
1 tbsp tamari
large pinch of ground black pepper
1 cauliflower, cut into florets
250 g/8¾ oz/3¾ cups kale or cavolo nero, roughly chopped
juice of 1 lemon
lemon wedges, to serve

1. Wash the lentils in a colander and leave to drain.

2. Heat a large lidded saucepan and add the coconut oil. Once melted, turn the heat down to low and add the onions, garlic, ginger and chilli. Leave to sauté for 5 minutes, until the onion is soft.

3. Add the spices and mix well. Remove 4 tablespoons of the mixture to garnish the bowls before serving. Add the leeks, carrots, celery and lentils and stir to coat with the onion mix.

4. Pour the bone broth or vegetable stock into the large saucepan and stir well.

5. Add the coriander/cilantro, tamari and pepper and stir well. Add the cauliflower. Cover and leave to simmer for a minimum of 30 minutes, stirring the bottom of the pan to prevent sticking.

6. Once the lentils and vegetables are cooked through, add the kale or cavolo nero and mix in with the lemon juice. Add more broth or water, if needed.

7. To serve, divide the dhal between bowls and add a spoonful of the onion mixture and a sprinkle of coriander/cilantro leaves to each, with a wedge of fresh lemon.

STICKY CHICKEN THIGHS

This is pure comfort food. I love these chicken thighs cooked on the barbecue in the summer with a crunchy fresh salad and a big spoon of guacamole or salsa. The kids love this with the Sweet Potato Wedges and Crispy Chickpea Bake (see page 191).

serves 4
140 g/5 oz tomato purée/paste
2 tbsp honey (optional)
1 tbsp tamari
1 tbsp apple cider vinegar
1 tsp paprika
generous pinch of black pepper
600 g/1 lb 5 oz organic chicken thighs
drizzle of rapeseed oil

for the salsa
4 large tomatoes
small handful of fresh coriander/cilantro,
    with stalks, finely chopped
1 green chilli, deseeded and finely chopped
1 small garlic clove, finely chopped
1 small red onion, finely chopped
juice of 1 lime
salt and ground black pepper, to season
drizzle of good-quality olive oil

1. Preheat the oven to 200°C/400°F/gas mark 6.

2. In a large bowl, mix together the tomato purée/paste, honey (if using), tamari, apple cider vinegar, paprika and pepper to make the marinade. Season to taste. Add the chicken thighs to the bowl and toss until each one is completely coated.

3. Put the thighs on a large baking tray. Drizzle with a little oil and bake for 20 minutes in the preheated oven, or until completely cooked through and golden brown. Turn halfway through cooking.

4. Meanwhile, make the salsa. Finely chop the tomatoes and add to a small bowl with the coriander/cilantro. Mix in the chilli, garlic, onion and lime juice. Season to taste and add a good glug of oil. Mix again and leave in the fridge until the chicken is ready.

5. Serve the thighs with sweet potato wedges, a green salad and a big spoonful of salsa.

LAMB KOFTAS WITH TOMATO AND ONION SALAD

Grass-fed lamb is packed with CLA (a naturally occurring fatty acid), which helps break down stored fats in the body. It can even help reduce inflammation in the gut.

serves 4

500 g/1 lb 2 oz organic minced/ground lamb
1 small onion, finely chopped
2 garlic cloves, crushed
1 fresh red chilli, deseeded and finely chopped
2-cm/¾-inch piece of fresh root ginger, peeled and grated
small handful of fresh mint leaves, chopped
small handful of coriander/cilantro leaves, chopped
½ tbsp ground cumin
½ tbsp ground coriander
1 tbsp tomato purée/paste
large pinch of Himalayan pink salt
4 tsp coconut oil, melted
lemon wedges, to serve

for the tomato and onion salad

4 tomatoes, chopped
1 red onion, chopped
4 fresh mint sprigs, chopped
2 fresh coriander/cilantro sprigs, chopped
1 tbsp olive oil
salt and ground black pepper, to season

1. Mix together the lamb, onion, garlic, chilli, ginger, herbs, spices, tomato purée/paste and salt in a bowl. Divide the mixture into 8 portions and roll each portion into a sausage shape. Thread each kofta onto a metal or bamboo skewer. Cover and keep in the fridge until you're ready to cook them.

2. To make the salad, mix the chopped tomatoes with the onion, mint, coriander/cilantro and olive oil. Season to taste.

3. Heat a griddle/grill pan over a medium heat. Lightly brush the koftas with the melted coconut oil. Cook them for 3–4 minutes on each side. Remove from the pan and serve with the Tomato and Onion Salad and a wedge of lemon.

Top Tip These koftas can be made in big batches and frozen. Just make sure you defrost them thoroughly before reheating.

MOROCCAN TAGINE

This is another one-pot lifesaver. Serve it with the Israeli salad from the Middle Eastern Bowl (see pages 128–129) and a big spoonful of quinoa. Cook a big batch and enjoy it throughout the week.

serves 4

1 butternut/winter squash (approximately 1.25 kg/2¾ lb), peeled and chopped into bite-sized chunks
salt and ground black pepper
1 tbsp coconut oil, melted
1 tbsp rapeseed oil
2 shallots, chopped
1 tsp ground cinnamon
3 garlic cloves, crushed
2 tbsp fresh root ginger, grated
2 red peppers, deseeded and sliced
2 aubergines/eggplants, chopped
1 x 400-g/14-oz can chickpeas, drained
1 x 400-g/14-oz can chopped tomatoes
400 ml/14 fl oz/1⅔ cups vegetable stock
4 tbsp fresh coriander/cilantro, chopped (stalks included)
1 tbsp ras el hanout
1½ tsp ground turmeric
1 tbsp Homemade Harissa (see page 185) or good-quality shop-bought

1. Preheat the oven to 180°C/350°F/gas mark 4 and line a baking tray with parchment paper.

2. Place the squash on the tray and drizzle with coconut oil. Season with salt and pepper. Roast in the preheated oven for 25 minutes, until cooked through.

3. Once the squash is nearly cooked, heat a large, lidded saucepan over a medium heat (or a tagine dish, if you are fancy) and add the rapeseed oil. Once hot, add the shallots, cinnamon, garlic and ginger. Leave to sauté for about 5 minutes.

4. Add the peppers, aubergines/eggplants and roasted squash and mix well. Then add the chickpeas, canned tomatoes, vegetable stock and the rest of the herbs and spices. Cover and leave to simmer for 20 minutes over a low heat. Season to taste.

TUNA POKE BOWL

One of my favourite restaurants is Granger & Co., which is lucky because it is less than a 30-second walk from Bodyism, London. As often as I can, I order their life-changing Tuna Poke dish; it is such a wholesome yet fresh-tasting meal. I've tried to make a simple version for you. The marinade is one of my favourites and works well with pretty much all fish.

serves 4

60 ml/2 fl oz/¼ cup tamari

1 tsp rice vinegar

1½ tsp sesame seeds (plus extra to garnish)

¾ tsp chilli flakes

4 spring onions/scallions, thinly sliced

450 g/1 lb/2¼ cups sushi-grade tuna, cut into 2-cm/¾-inch cubes

380 g/13½ oz/2 cups brown rice, cooked in stock

2 tomatoes, chopped

1 avocado, sliced lengthways

small handful of fresh coriander/cilantro, chopped

small handful of toasted coconut flakes

1. Mix the tamari, rice vinegar, sesame seeds, chilli flakes and spring onions/scallions in a bowl. Add the tuna and mix well. Leave to marinate for a minimum of 2 hours in the fridge or ideally overnight.

2. All you need to do is build your poke bowl. Spoon an equal amount of the rice into 4 bowls, add the tomatoes, a few slices of avocado and the tuna. Sprinkle with coriander/cilantro and coconut flakes and serve.

MIDDLE EASTERN MEATBALLS

The key to these meatballs is to finely mince all the ingredients with a sharp knife; this not only forms a smoother textured meatball, but also ensures they cook through evenly. Don't hold back with the herbs and spices — be guided by your own taste buds and choose whatever you like.

serves 4

450 g/1 lb minced/ground lamb or turkey
½ tsp ground cumin
¼ tsp ground coriander
1 garlic clove, crushed
half a small red onion, finely minced
1 tsp chilli, finely minced
handful of fresh coriander/cilantro, finely chopped
handful of fresh parsley, finely chopped
1 organic, free-range egg, lightly beaten
1 tsp olive oil
1 x 400-g/14-oz can chopped tomatoes
1 tsp salt
1 tsp ground black pepper
½ tsp ground sumac
5–6 whole cabbage leaves, to serve

1. Put the meat, ground cumin, ground coriander, garlic, chilli, chopped herbs and beaten egg in a bowl. Using clean hands, mix everything together and ensure the flavourings are well distributed.

2. Again using your hands, or a big spoon, roll the mixture into medium-sized balls (you should get 7–8 meatballs).

3. Heat the olive oil in a large frying pan/skillet over a high heat and place the meatballs in; you should hear a good sizzle when you do this.

4. Brown the meatballs for 1 minute on each side. If you feel the meat has released a lot of fat into the pan, take the meatballs out, discard the fat and put the meatballs back in.

5. Once your meatballs are brown on all sides, pour in the tomatoes and add the salt, pepper and sumac.

6. Leave the meatballs in the tomato sauce to simmer and finish cooking for about 7 minutes. You can check if they're done by cutting into one or by pressing the meat with a finger (the meatball should feel quite firm).

7. While the meatballs are cooking, prepare the cabbage leaves. I find the easiest way is to chop the bottom root off the cabbage and pull the whole leaves off one by one.

8. Wrap each meatball, with a drizzle of sauce, in a cabbage leaf and enjoy!

SEXY STIR-FRY

We all need a dish that we can rustle up when there is nothing left in the fridge. This is so simple, delicious, healthy and quick. Use up whatever veg you have lying around — it doesn't have to be the combination listed below. Add prawns/shrimp or thinly sliced chicken to increase the protein. The eggs make this meal more substantial; if you don't want them scrambled, serve them fried, on top of the noodles, with a few coriander/cilantro leaves and a grind of fresh pepper.

serves 4

200 g/7 oz flat, wide rice noodles
2 tbsp tamari or soy sauce
½ tbsp honey
1½ tbsp freshly squeezed lime juice, plus an extra squeeze, to serve
1 tbsp coconut or vegetable or olive oil, plus extra for scrambling the eggs
1 carrot, peeled and finely sliced into discs
1 red or yellow pepper, finely sliced lengthways
1 small courgette/zucchini, peeled and finely sliced into discs
1 tsp finely minced fresh chilli, or dried chilli flakes
2 garlic cloves, finely minced
1 tsp finely minced fresh root ginger
2 organic, free-range eggs, whisked
1 tbsp sesame seeds
handful of fresh coriander/cilantro, roughly chopped

1. First, soak the noodles in a bowl of hot water; they can soften while you get the rest of the ingredients ready. They should soften up in under 10 minutes.

2. Mix the tamari, honey and lime juice in a bowl.

3. Put a large frying pan/skillet over a high heat and pour in the oil. Let it heat up and then throw in the carrots to cook for a minute, followed by the peppers. Let them sauté and get some colour for about 2 minutes on the high heat and then add in the courgette/zucchini, the chilli (if using fresh), garlic and ginger. Stir everything around and cook for 2 minutes.

4. Now pour over the tamari, honey and lime juice sauce and mix everything together well.

5. Transfer everything from the pan to a plate or bowl.

6. Drain the noodles.

7. Add a small splash of oil to the pan and pour in the whisked eggs with a pinch of salt and pepper (remember the tamari/soy is salty).

8. Whisk the eggs and, when they start to scramble, add the noodles and stir them into the egg mixture.

9. Add the rest of your ingredients back in, mix everything together, adding your dried chilli flakes now, if using.

10. Add a final squeeze of lime, the sesame seeds, coriander/cilantro, and serve.

SLOW-COOKED IRISH STEW

This dish is not only comforting and hearty, it is also really healthy and a great cold-buster. Stews are about building layers of flavour, so take the time to do each step properly and enjoy the process. Get organized and prep your vegetables and garlic beforehand — then it's super simple.

serves 4

1 tbsp olive oil
700 g/1½ lb lamb neck, cubed
1 white onion, finely minced
2 large garlic cloves, finely minced
3 carrots, peeled and chopped
1 large parsnip, peeled and chopped
large handful of cavolo nero or kale,
    chopped (stalks discarded)
2 bay leaves
a few sprigs of thyme
1 rosemary stalk
½ tsp salt
½ tsp ground black pepper
5 baby potatoes, chopped (optional)

1. Preheat the oven to 180°C/350°F/gas mark 4.

2. First comes browning the meat, which gives colour and seals in flavour. In a big, lidded casserole dish or pot, heat half of the olive oil over a high heat. Add in the meat. If there isn't enough room in your pot for each meat piece to have contact with the bottom of the pan to brown, do it in batches. Do the first side for 2 minutes and then turn. You should hear a good sizzle when the meat hits the pan.

3. Once browned, take all the meat out of the pot and set aside. Turn down the heat to medium and add in the rest of the olive oil.

4. Add in the onion and stir. Try to scrape up any brown bits at the bottom of the pan from the meat, because these are full of flavour. Once the onion is translucent, after about 2 minutes, add in the garlic and cook for another minute.

5. Add in the chopped carrots, parsnip, kale, bay leaves and herbs and add half the salt and pepper. Stir everything together.

6. Put all the meat back in the pot and pour in enough boiling water to cover the meat.

7. Add the remaining salt and pepper and stir everything together. If using the potatoes, let them just rest on top of the meat and water. Put a lid on the pot and put it into the preheated oven for at least 2½ hours, or 3 if you have the time.

8. Serve up into bowls and enjoy.

MIRACLE BONE BROTH

This incredible bone broth is packed with antioxidants and collagen, making it a truly healthy elixir. You can use leftover bones from a Sunday roast or ask the butcher — often they'll give them to you for free! Ensure you're using collagen-rich bones, like marrow, knuckles and feet, from organic lamb or chicken.

This recipe has a few steps, but nothing complicated and the result is so worth it. It also makes quite a bit of broth, so you can freeze some and keep the rest in your fridge for up to 4 days. Feel free to drink a cup on its own or add it to curries, pasta sauces and use as a stock base for soups for a nutritional boost.

Start your broth in the morning — you'll want to leave it simmering over a low heat for up to 12 hours to get maximum nourishment from the bones. At room temperature, it has a jelly-like consistency. If it looks strange — you've made it correctly.

---

serves 4, with leftovers

1 kg/2¼ lb organic lamb or chicken bones (marrow, knuckles, feet or other collagen-rich bones)
3 onions, skin on, chopped in half
3 carrots, chopped in half
5 garlic cloves, smashed
4 bay leaves
½ tbsp peppercorns
½ tsp salt
½ tbsp apple cider vinegar

1. Preheat the oven to 200°C/400°F/gas mark 6.

2. Put the bones in a large pot and fill with cold water; bring this up to the boil over a high heat and let it boil for about 20 minutes. This initial step removes all the impurities from the bones and is called blanching.

3. Discard the water, put the bones in a roasting tin and place in the oven to caramelize for about an hour. This enhances the depth of flavour in the broth and starts breaking down the collagen in the bones.

4. Return the bones to your pot, together with the onions, carrots, garlic, bay leaves, peppercorns, salt and cider vinegar, and refill with (preferably filtered) water. These few additional ingredients add an aromatic quality to your broth and really deepen the flavour.

5. Bring up to the boil, then turn down and leave to simmer for as long as you can — preferably up to 12 hours to really get the maximum nutrition out of the bones and develop a flavoursome broth.

6. To finish, pour the broth through a fine-mesh sieve/strainer into a wide and shallow container, which will help the broth cool down quicker. All the fat will rise to the top once the broth cools; skim the fat off and either discard it or use it for other recipes.

7. Once cool, refrigerate or freeze.

POACHED COCONUT CHICKEN AND CAULI-RICE

This is a quick, easy and fuss-free dinner. If using a box grater for the cauliflower, do it on top of the baking sheet in which you plan to roast it to save on mess.

serves 2

2 organic chicken breasts (approximately 150 g/5¼ oz each)
1 head of cauliflower
¼ tsp salt
¼ tsp ground black pepper
½ tbsp coconut oil, melted
1 lemongrass stalk
1 x 400-ml/14-fl oz can coconut milk
half a small red chilli
2-cm/¾-inch piece of fresh root ginger
½ tbsp fish sauce
1 red or yellow pepper, julienned
handful of fresh coriander/cilantro, chopped
juice of 1 lime

1. Preheat the oven to 190°C/375°F/gas mark 5.

2. Let the chicken come to room temperature while you prepare the other ingredients.

3. Either grate the whole head of cauliflower with a box grater or place it in a food processor and pulse to small rice-sized pieces. Sprinkle with half the salt and pepper and pour over the coconut oil.

4. Mix with your hands and spread thinly on a baking sheet. Put into the preheated oven and leave to roast for 20 minutes. After about 10 minutes, give it a toss.

5. Bash the lemongrass stalk with the back of a spoon a few times to bruise it and release its aroma. Pour the coconut milk into a medium–hot pan and add the lemongrass, chilli, ginger and fish sauce. Let it simmer for approximately 3 minutes.

6. Sprinkle both chicken breasts with the remaining salt and pepper. Add the chicken and sliced pepper to the pan of simmering sauce. Turn both breasts after 5 minutes and do the same again 5 minutes later. The chicken should be cooked in just under 15 minutes.

7. Take the chicken out and cover in tin foil. Turn up the heat in the pan and boil the sauce to reduce and thicken it for about 3 minutes. Shred the chicken with a fork and add it back into the flavoursome sauce.

8. Divide the cauli-rice between two plates and spoon the chicken on top. Sprinkle over the chopped coriander/cilantro and add a final squeeze of lime.

KERALAN FISH CURRY

The subtle heat in this dish comes from the green chilli and ginger, while the spices bring a warm depth to the dish that is hard to describe but it is absolutely delicious.

serves 4, with leftovers

for the masala

1 tbsp coriander seeds

1 tsp cumin seeds

2 star anise

1 tsp ground turmeric

3 garlic cloves, finely minced

half a small green chilli, deseeded and chopped

1 tsp salt

2.5-cm/1-inch piece of fresh root ginger, peeled and grated or finely minced

for the dish

1½ tbsp vegetable, coconut or olive oil

1 red onion, finely chopped

1 large tomato, chopped into small chunks

½ tsp white vinegar

100 ml/3½ fl oz/hot water

1 x 400-ml/14-fl oz can coconut milk

400 g/14 oz firm white fish, like cod or pollock, cut into even-sized chunks

200 g/7 oz prawns/shrimp

¼ tsp freshly ground black pepper

pinch of salt

juice of half a lime

large handful of fresh coriander/cilantro, roughly chopped

1. Make the masala first. Toast the spices in a hot, dry pan to release their flavours. Grind the spices into a powder in a food processor or coffee grinder and mix in the garlic, chilli, salt and ginger.

2. Heat 1 tablespoon of oil in a medium–hot frying pan/skillet and sauté the onion for about 2 minutes, until softened. Add in the masala paste and let it cook for a few minutes, until you can really smell the spices, and the garlic, ginger and chilli are cooked.

3. Add in the chopped tomatoes and the vinegar and let everything cook in the pan for a minute.

4. Add the hot water and let the whole mix simmer for about 5 minutes.

5. If you're making brown rice or quinoa to accompany this dish, now is the time to get it going in another pot. Follow the packet instructions and, if cooking quinoa, be sure to put a lid on the pot to properly cook the grain and, once done, cover with a tea/dish towel to allow it to continue steaming. This makes for light, airy quinoa.

6. After 5 minutes of the masala mix simmering, add in the can of coconut milk and stir everything together.

7. Add in the fish, prawns/shrimp, pepper and salt. Simmer for about 7 minutes, until the fish is cooked.

8. Squeeze the lime juice into the pan and toss in the coriander/cilantro. Taste the sauce to see if it needs more lime, salt or pepper. Serve up with brown rice, quinoa or your grains of choice!

PERFECT ROAST CHICKEN

Everyone needs a roast chicken recipe up their sleeve. It is truly one of the most delicious, nourishing and comforting meals ever, and will see you through so many dinners and special occasions. It's worth investing in a beautiful, organic, free-range bird; yes, it's more expensive, but one chicken can stretch into two or three meals. Not only will you have leftovers, but you can turn the carcass into delicious and healthy stock to make tasty soups (see page 167), pasta sauces... the list goes on.

serves 4

1 tsp olive oil
1 x 1.9-kg/4-lb 3 oz chicken
½ tsp ground Himalayan pink salt
½ tsp freshly ground black pepper
half a lemon
half an onion
a few garlic cloves, smashed
a few sprigs of thyme or rosemary (use whichever herbs you have)

1. Preheat the oven to 200°C/400°F/gas mark 6 and allow at least 15 minutes for it to heat up properly.

2. Pour the olive oil over the chicken and sprinkle with the salt and pepper, including the cavity. Using your hands, rub the seasoning into the chicken skin.

3. Put the lemon, onion, garlic and herbs into the chicken cavity. This will give the chicken a lovely flavour as it cooks.

4. Put the chicken into a roasting dish and cook in the preheated oven for 1 hour.

5. Take the chicken out, baste with the liquid that's in the bottom of the pan and cover with tin foil.

6. Allow it to rest for at least 10 minutes; this lets all the juices go back into the chicken, making the bird tender and delicious.

7. Use this time, while the chicken rests, to crisp up any vegetables you have roasting or to prepare a salad. Slice, serve and enjoy.

Top Tip If you're making stock, just simmer the chicken carcass in a large pot of water with any vegetable scraps and herbs you have in the fridge and plenty of salt and pepper for 2 hours — it's so simple and satisfying.

CHICKEN SCHNITZEL WITH ROOT VEGETABLE MASH

Who said healthy food couldn't include comfort food? This is such a warming, hearty and healthy dinner and it's one of our favourites. Enjoy it with some delicious wholegrain mustard and a side of sautéed greens.

serves 2

for the mash

190 g/6⅔ oz/1⅓ cups butternut/winter squash, chopped
1 tbsp coconut oil, melted
half a cauliflower, chopped (you can use the stalk)
120 ml/4 fl oz/½ cup almond milk
3 garlic cloves, crushed
1 tbsp wholegrain mustard
Himalayan pink salt and ground black pepper, to season

for the schnitzel

2 tbsp arrowroot flour
2 tbsp chickpea/gram flour
1 tsp garlic powder
1 organic, free-range egg, beaten
2 small organic chicken breasts (approximately 150 g/5¼ oz each)
1 tbsp coconut oil

1. Preheat the oven to 180°C/350°F/gas mark 4 and line a baking tray with parchment paper.

2. Place the chopped squash on the baking tray and drizzle with oil. Roast in the oven for 30 minutes.

3. Meanwhile, steam the cauliflower for 5 minutes or until it is very tender.

4. In a food processor, blend the roasted squash, almond milk, crushed garlic cloves and cauliflower. Stir in the wholegrain mustard and season well.

5. For the schnitzel, mix the flours together with a pinch of salt and pepper and the garlic powder. Divide the flour mixture into two bowls. Pour the egg into a third.

6. Cover a work surface with a piece of clingfilm/plastic wrap. Place the chicken breasts on top and cover with another piece of clingfilm/plastic wrap. Using a rolling pin, bash each chicken breast until they are approximately 3-mm/⅛-inch thick.

7. Dip the chicken into the flour to coat and then dip it into the egg mix and then into the last bowl of flour to coat, ensuring an even layer on each side.

8. Put the mash into a saucepan and cook over a low heat, until warm and ready to serve.

9. Heat the coconut oil a large frying pan/skillet over a medium–high heat. When the oil is really hot, fry the chicken for 3 minutes, until crisp and crunchy on the underside. Carefully turn it and cook for another 2–3 minutes, until cooked through. Serve the schnitzel with the mash and sautéed greens.

THE PERFECT BURGER

There are three secrets to the perfect burger. The first is to ensure the garlic and onion are really finely chopped, so they mix well with the meat and cook through properly. The second is to ensure your meat mixture isn't too wet, or else the burgers won't hold together. When adding the egg, pour in half of it first and mix with your hands; if the mixture feels like it will come together and form nice patties, then leave the other half of the whisked egg out. The third is to ensure you have properly seasoned the raw mince for fantastic flavour. Now, go on, steal my secrets and make a damn tasty burger!

serves 4

1 garlic clove, finely chopped
handful of finely chopped red onion
handful of fresh parsley, finely chopped
500 g/1 lb 2 oz minced/ground lamb
½ tsp salt
½ tsp ground black pepper
½ tbsp Dijon or wholegrain mustard
1 organic, free-range egg, beaten
½ tbsp olive oil

1. Add the minced garlic, onion and parsley to a bowl with the meat. Season the meat with the salt and black pepper.

2. Add the mustard and pour in half the beaten egg. Mix it all together with your hands and judge whether the mix could do with more egg or if it will form firm burger patties without it.

3. Form the mixture into 4 large burger patties or 6 smaller ones (bear in mind that the smaller ones will take less time to cook).

4. Heat up a large frying pan/skillet over a high heat and, once hot, add the oil. Let it get hot (this will take 1–2 minutes).

5. Add the burgers to the pan; you should hear a sizzle when you do this — if not, the pan isn't hot enough and the burgers will taste bland. Sear the burgers for about 4 minutes on each side. Test the meat with your finger; it should feel firm and a little springy to the touch for medium doneness. You could finish them in a hot oven for another few minutes, if you like your meat well done, but I think this dries the burgers out and ruins the texture.

6. Take off the heat and leave to rest for 1–2 minutes before serving; this allows all the juices to run back into the middle of the burger, keeping it moist and juicy — enjoy!

LEFTOVER ROAST CHICKEN PHO

I always make this after we've had a roast, because it's a delicious way of using up leftovers. The tangy flavours of the tamari and brown-rice miso are so tasty. If you want an extra protein boost, enjoy it with a soft-boiled egg!

serves 4

1 whole organic corn-fed, free-range chicken carcass (it's best to make this soup after you make Perfect Roast Chicken, on page 162)

500 ml/17 fl oz/2 cups organic chicken stock

1 whole red chilli

thumb of fresh root ginger, grated

1 lemongrass stalk, bashed

1 tbsp tamari

1 tbsp organic apple cider vinegar

1 tbsp brown-rice miso paste

1 tbsp fish sauce

225 g/8 oz buckwheat soba noodles

150 g/5¼ oz/1½ cups sugar snap peas

200 g/7 oz/3 cups mushrooms, sliced

4 tbsp spring onions/scallions, thinly sliced

4 tbsp fresh coriander/cilantro, roughly chopped, to garnish

1. In a large stockpot, combine the chicken carcass with the chicken stock, bring to the boil and simmer over a low heat for at least 1 hour. Remove from the heat; the remaining chicken meat should have fallen off the bone. Strain through a sieve/strainer and discard the bones, returning the meat to the reserved liquid. Put back over a low heat and add the chilli, ginger, lemongrass, tamari, vinegar, brown-rice miso and fish sauce. Simmer while you prepare the soba noodles.

2. Cook the soba noodles according to the packet instructions, keeping them on the al dente side. When they are cooked, rinse them immediately with cold water; this will prevent them getting soggy.

3. Add the sugar snap peas and mushrooms to the stockpot and simmer for 15 minutes.

4. To serve, distribute the soba noodles into 4 soup bowls and top with ladles of the stock. Garnish with spring onions/scallions and fresh coriander/cilantro.

PRAWN SUMMER ROLLS WITH TAMARI DIPPING SAUCE

These rolls are such a delicious appetizer for a dinner party. If you want to get really fancy, buy some edible flowers to add into the roll. As always, use this recipe as a guide and feel free to experiment. Swap the prawns/shrimp for chicken or more vegetables; choose whatever makes you happy!

makes 10

1 tsp butter or olive oil
1 garlic clove, crushed
10 fresh king prawns/jumbo shrimp
10 rice paper rolls
half a cucumber, cut lengthways and finely sliced lengthways
1 whole red pepper, finely sliced lengthways
3 spring onions/scallions, finely sliced lengthways
5 radishes, finely sliced
handful of fresh coriander/cilantro, chopped
juice of 2 limes

for the dipping sauce

5 tbsp tamari
3 tbsp tahini
juice of 1 lemon
salt and ground black pepper, to taste

1. Heat the butter or oil over a medium heat in a small frying pan/skillet. Add the garlic and the prawns/shrimp and fry until golden on both sides; this takes 5–10 minutes. Remove from the heat and set aside. Slice each prawn/shrimp in half, so you have 20 prawn/shrimp halves to put in the rolls.

2. Fill a large bowl with boiling hot water and dip the first rice paper roll into it, until it is translucent.

3. Put the roll on a plate and put 2 prawn/shrimp halves face down on top, with 3 pieces each of cucumber, pepper, spring onion/scallion and radish.

4. Garnish with 1 teaspoon of coriander/cilantro and drizzle ¼ teaspoon of lime juice over the top.

5. Fold the outer edges in and roll into a small parcel.

6. Repeat for all the rolls.

7. To make the dipping sauce, combine all the ingredients in a small jug/pitcher and mix until well combined. Pour into a bowl to dip the rolls in.

SNACKS AND SIDES

PISTACHIO AND RASPBERRY MEDICINE BALLS

I really don't like when energy balls are marketed as 'healthy' but are filled with loads of 'fake' sugars. That's why I try to experiment with other ways of sweetening our energy balls — things like pumpkin or berries, or good fats like coconut butter or nut butter. This ingredient list makes me smile, because it's full of nourishing, wonderful ingredients.

makes 20

150 g/5¼ oz/1 cup almonds
20 g/¾ oz coconut oil, melted
200 g/7 oz/¾ cup frozen raspberries
20 g/¾ oz chia seeds
2 tbsp almond butter
100 g/3½ oz/1⅓ cups desiccated/dried shredded coconut (plus extra, for sprinkling)
50 g/1¾ oz/⅓ cup hemp seeds
50 g/1¾ oz/⅓ cup buckwheat groats
1 scoop Bodyism Protein Excellence
100 g/3½ oz/⅔ cup raw chocolate (optional, for dipping)

1. Put the almonds in a food processor and blend into a breadcrumb texture. Add the rest of the ingredients and blend until everything is well combined.

2. Use your hands to roll the mixture into walnut-sized balls.

3. Roll the balls in the coconut, then place in an airtight container and stick them in the freezer for a minimum of 30 minutes. Enjoy them straight out of the freezer.

4. If you want to make these extra indulgent, melt some raw chocolate and dip the balls in the chocolate before placing them in the freezer.

TRAIL MIX

This is my go-to when I'm travelling. I don't know what it is about flying, but I'm always hungry on the plane. This very easy Trail Mix is an easy way to keep satisfied and happy during your travels. Also, it's a great topping for the Açai Bowl (see page 96), Protein Pancakes (see page 105) or Three-Grain Porridge (see page 100).

makes 500 g/1 lb 2 oz

2 tbsp coconut oil
2½ tsp vanilla powder
200 g/7 oz/1½ cups almonds
50 g/1¾ oz/½ cup pumpkin seeds
50 g/1¾ oz/⅔ cup coconut flakes
100 g/3½ oz/1 cup flaked/slivered almonds
50 g/1¾ oz/⅓ cup mulberries
50 g/1¾ oz/½ cup goji berries or dark/
   bittersweet chocolate chips

1. Preheat the oven to 180°C/350°F/gas mark 4 and line a baking tray with parchment paper.

2. Melt the coconut oil and stir in the vanilla powder.

3. Place the almonds, pumpkin seeds, coconut flakes and flaked/slivered almonds in a bowl and mix in the melted coconut oil and vanilla. Stir until everything is covered.

4. Pour the mix onto the lined baking tray, place in the preheated oven and bake for about 20 minutes, until the almonds have got darker and the coconut flakes have turned golden brown.

5. Once cooked, take the mix out of the oven, leave to cool and then stir in the mulberries and goji berries/ dark/bittersweet chocolate chips.

6. Place in an airtight container and enjoy whenever you need a healthy snack on the go.

PECAN SALTED CHOCOLATE BARK

I always thought making my own chocolate wouldn't be worth the fuss, but this recipe is so simple and makes a much tastier treat than any shop-bought one. It's also perfect for wrapping up and giving as a healthy gift. I like to play around with flavour combinations, but the Pecan Salted Chocolate Bark is always my favourite.

serves 4

100 g/3½ oz/1 cup pecans
½ tbsp coconut oil
150 ml/5¼ fl oz/⅔ cup maple syrup
1 tbsp ground cinnamon
150 g/5¼ oz/¾ cup cacao butter
85 g/3 oz/¾ cup raw cacao powder
2 pinches of sea salt flakes

1. Preheat the oven to 150°C/300°F/gas mark 2 and line 2 baking tins with parchment paper. Pour the pecans into the first tin.

2. Meanwhile, melt the coconut oil in a saucepan over a low heat with 50 ml/2 fl oz/¼ cup of the maple syrup and the cinnamon, stirring until well combined.

3. Pour the mixture over the pecans and mix until all the pecans are covered. Pop them into the preheated oven for 10 minutes, until they are golden.

4. Melt the cacao butter in a bowl set over boiling water; make sure the bowl isn't touching the water, and stir until completely melted. Take off the heat and rest.

5. Mix the cacao powder into the melted cacao butter and keep stirring for 3–4 minutes, until the mixture thickens up — this is the most important part of the recipe, so keep at it until it feels thick and has the consistency of melted chocolate.

6. Pour the chocolate mixture into the second baking tin, so it's about 1-cm/½-inch thick. Sprinkle the pecans into the chocolate, pressing them down to make sure they are completely set into it. Sprinkle sea salt on top and place in the freezer for 2 hours.

7. Take the chocolate out and break it up into sections, however big or small you like. I keep my chocolate in the freezer in an airtight container, because it retains all the flavour and has a semifreddo-type consistency. However, keeping it in the fridge is perfectly fine, too.

NOT-ELLA

You all know about my Nutella addiction. This is my healthier version, which Chrissy has to hide when it's in the house — otherwise my addiction might reappear and you'll find me in a bath of healthy nut butter...

makes 1 jar
250 g/8¾ oz/1⅔ cups raw hazelnuts
2 tbsp water
2 tbsp maple syrup (optional)
1 tbsp cacao powder
1 tsp vanilla extract
½ tsp sea salt
2 tbsp cacao nibs

1. Preheat the oven to 180°C/350°F/gas mark 4.

2. Place the hazelnuts on a baking tray and leave to roast for 5–7 minutes, until toasted. Remove and leave to cool.

3. Place the hazelnuts in a food processor and whizz on medium speed for about 10 minutes, until a paste forms. Stop every few minutes to scrape the nuts from the blade.

4. Add the remaining ingredients (apart from the cacao nibs) and pulse for a few more minutes.

5. Sprinkle the cacao nibs on top so that when you transfer the mixture to a jar they are distributed throughout. Enjoy!

BODYISM COOKIES

These cookies have their own fan club. When we've run out of them at our café in West London, protests have started. Seriously, these cookies are pretty damn good. That's why I've given you a recipe that makes 18, because they disappear before your very eyes. If you want to be smart, freeze half of the dough and, when you fancy another batch, just defrost and roll it out. Drum roll, please...

makes 18–20

120 g/4¼ oz/1⅓ cups oat flour (or gluten-free oats blitzed to a fine powder in a food processor)

60 g/2 oz/½ cup coconut flour

180 g/6⅓ oz/2¼ cups gluten-free oats

½ tsp bicarbonate of soda/baking soda

225 g/8 oz/1cup plus 2 tbsp coconut palm sugar

1 tsp Himalayan pink salt

2 tsp vanilla extract

150 g/5¼ oz/¾ cup coconut oil, melted

3 organic, free-range eggs, beaten

100 g/3½ oz/⅔ cup sugar-free dark/bittersweet chocolate, cut into small squares

1. Preheat the oven to 200°C/400°F/gas mark 6 and line 2 baking trays with parchment paper.

2. In a large mixing bowl, mix the flours, oats, bicarbonate of soda/baking soda, sugar and salt together.

3. In another bowl, mix the vanilla extract and coconut oil together.

4. Slowly mix the liquid mixture into the dry mixture. Then slowly stir in the beaten eggs.

5. Finally, add the chocolate, and, using your hands, mix it in.

6. Roll 1 dessertspoon of the cookie dough into a small ball and place on a baking tray. Repeat this step until you've used up all the mixture, making sure you leave quite a bit of space between each ball.

7. Using the back of a fork, flatten each ball.

8. Bake in the oven for 12–15 minutes, until golden brown. Then leave to cool (remember they cook more as they cool down).

ALMOND BUTTER JAM MUFFINS

Muffins can be the most delicious, indulgent snack in the world — or the biggest disappointment. These muffins are really gooey and the almond butter and jam give them the perfect balance of salt and sweet.

makes 12

100 g/3½ oz/1 cup pecans
2 organic, free-range eggs, beaten
90 ml/3 fl oz/⅓ cup maple syrup
50 g/1¾ oz/¼ cup coconut palm sugar
60 ml/2 fl oz/¼ cup coconut oil, melted
190 g/6⅔ oz/¾ cup apple sauce
130 g/4½ oz/½ cup almond butter
pinch of sea salt
1½ tsp baking powder
½ tsp bicarbonate of soda/baking soda
1 tsp apple cider vinegar
60 ml/2 fl oz/¼ cup almond milk
50 g/1¾ oz/½ cup quinoa flour
50 g/1¾ oz/½ cup buckwheat flour
50 g/1¾ oz/½ cup ground almonds
60 g/2 oz/¾ cup gluten-free oats
6 tsp sugar-free strawberry jam

1. Preheat the oven to 180°C/350°F/gas mark 4 and line a standard muffin tin with 12 muffin cases.

2. Pour the eggs into a mixing bowl, add the maple syrup, coconut sugar and oil and whisk well.

3. Add the apple sauce, almond butter, salt, baking powder, bicarbonate of soda/baking soda, apple cider vinegar and whisk to combine.

4. Add the almond milk and whisk again to combine.

5. Lastly, add the flours, ground almonds and oats and whisk or stir until just combined.

6. Spoon the mixture into the muffin cases until they are half full. Then add half a teaspoon of sugar-free strawberry jam to each. Add a tablespoon more mixture on top of the jam, to cover it.

7. Place in the preheated oven and cook for 25 minutes, until a cocktail stick/toothpick inserted into the centre of one of the muffins comes out clean.

BODYISM BANANA MUFFINS

The flour mix that we use in this recipe is our go-to for any cake. The different flours make the perfect gluten-free replacement for starchy plain flour. Just mix it up and then keep the leftovers to make any other gluten-free cake that takes your fancy.

makes 12

155 g/1 cup plus 2 tbsp gluten-free flour mix
 (see below)
6 tbsp almond flour
1 tsp baking powder
¾ tsp Himalayan pink salt
½ tsp ground cinnamon
3 tbsp linseeds/flaxseeds
3 tbsp roughly chopped walnuts, toasted
6 tbsp coconut oil, melted
6 tbsp maple syrup
6 tbsp coconut milk
2 tbsp almond butter
2 tsp vanilla extract
6 ripe bananas (4 mashed, 2 sliced)

for the gluten-free flour mix

440 g/15½ oz/2¾ cups brown rice flour
160 g/5⅔ oz/1¾ cups oat flour (or gluten-
 free oats blitzed to a fine powder in a food
 processor)
200 g/7 oz/1¾ cups coconut flour
60 g/2 oz/½ cup tapioca flour

1. Preheat the oven to 180°C/350°F/gas mark 4 and line a 12-cup muffin tin with 12 paper liners or 2 x 6-cup muffin tins with 6 paper liners each.

2. In a large bowl, mix together the flour mix, almond flour, baking powder, salt, cinnamon and linseeds/flaxseeds to remove any lumps. Stir in the walnuts.

3. In a small bowl, combine the oil, 5 tablespoons of the maple syrup, the coconut milk, almond butter and vanilla. Whisk to combine. Fold in the mashed bananas.

4. Pour the wet mixture into the dry mixture and whisk together by hand, until just combined.

5. Lightly toss the sliced bananas with the remaining maple syrup.

6. Fill the muffin cups almost all the way up and top with 3 banana slices per muffin.

7. Bake for 35–40 minutes in the preheated oven, until the muffins have browned and spring back slightly to the touch.

Top Tip Whenever you eat fruit, try to eat it with a good fat, because it slows down the absorption of the sugar so that you don't have a sugar spike and become moody for the rest of the afternoon.

HUMMUS WITH HARISSA AND ROASTED CARROT DIPPERS

This is quite simply the most delicious hummus ever made (not that I'm confident or anything). The baking soda does something magical to the chickpeas to make a creamy, smooth finish every time. The homemade harissa gives it a fiery kick, which is perfect with the sweetness of the roasted carrot dippers. Although soaking dried chickpeas may seem like a laborious process, you will thank me when you try the end result.

serves 4
2 tablespoons Homemade Harissa (see page 185)

for the hummus
250 g/8¾ oz/1¼ cups dried chickpeas
1 tsp bicarbonate of soda/baking soda
270 g/9½ oz/1 cup plus 2 tbsp tahini paste
4 garlic cloves, crushed
pinch of salt and ground black pepper
4 tbsp freshly squeezed lemon juice
100 ml/3½ fl oz ice-cold water

for the roasted carrot dippers
2 bunches of baby carrots, scrubbed clean
1–2 tbsp olive oil
salt

1. Begin by making the hummus. Put the chickpeas in a large bowl and cover with double the volume of cold water. Leave to soak overnight.

2. The next day, drain the chickpeas and transfer to a saucepan. Add 1 teaspoon of baking soda and cook over a low heat for 3–4 minutes, stirring constantly.

3. Add 1.5 litres/2⅔ pints/6 cups of cold water to the pan, bring to the boil and gently simmer the chickpeas, skimming off any foam or skins that float to the top. This can take 20–40 minutes. They are ready when you can press a chickpea between finger and thumb and it breaks gently. Check the firmness every 10 minutes.

4. Drain the chickpeas and blitz in a food processor until you achieve a smooth paste. Then, with the food processor still running, add the tahini, crushed garlic, salt, pepper and lemon juice. Slowly drizzle in the ice-cold water until you get a smooth, creamy paste. Transfer into a bowl and let it rest for at least 30 minutes before serving.

5. To make the carrot dippers, first preheat the oven to 180°C/350°F/gas mark 4. On a baking sheet, drizzle the carrots with 1–2 tablespoons of olive oil and then toss. Sprinkle with salt. Roast for 20 minutes, until browned on the bottom and cooked through. Remove and set aside. Enjoy cool, with the harissa drizzled over them, and with the hummus for dipping.

GUACAMOLE

I love smashed avo... as does the rest of the world, these days. This is my fail-safe smashed avo recipe, which can be varied depending on what you are pairing it with. Try adding chilli flakes, or fresh sprigs of mint, or finely chopped pepper. The options are endless!

serves 4

2 avocados

1 garlic clove, peeled and crushed

1 large tomato, deseeded and chopped

juice of half a lemon

half a red chilli, deseeded and finely
    chopped

small handful of fresh coriander/cilantro,
    chopped

generous pinch of salt

1. Mash the avocados in a bowl and mix in the garlic, chopped tomato, lemon juice, chilli, coriander/cilantro and salt.

ROSEMARY PARSNIP FRIES

Parsnips are the perfect winter alternative to French fries, and the rosemary and garlic in this recipe add a flavourful punch.

serves 4

4 large parsnips

1 tbsp olive oil

¼ tsp salt

¼ tsp ground black pepper

1 garlic clove, crushed

3 rosemary stalks

1. Preheat the oven to 190°C/375°F/gas mark 5.

2. Peel and cut the parsnips into long French-fry-like pieces.

3. Scatter the parsnips on a roasting pan.

4. Pour over the olive oil, sprinkle on the salt, pepper and garlic, and lay the rosemary sprigs on top.

5. Roast the parsnips in the preheated oven for 10 minutes, then carefully turn them and return to the oven for a further 10–15 minutes.

MUHAMMARA (ROASTED RED PEPPER DIP)

I love travelling to Turkey, partly because it's beautiful (our gym at the D-Hotel is one of the most stunning places that I've been lucky enough to visit), but also because I love Turkish cuisine. This dip was inspired by my travels there and it makes crudités way more interesting.

serves 4

3 large red peppers
80 g/2¾ oz/¾ cup walnuts, toasted (plus a few extra, to serve)
3 tbsp olive oil (plus extra, to serve)
120 ml/4¼ oz/½ cup water
small handful of fresh coriander/cilantro leaves, chopped (plus extra, to serve)
1 tbsp apple cider vinegar
half a garlic clove, peeled

1. Preheat the oven to 180°C/350°F/gas mark 4 and line a baking tray with parchment paper.

2. Cut the peppers in half, remove the seeds, and place on the baking tray. Roast in the preheated oven for 20 minutes, until slightly blackened. Leave to cool.

3. Once cool, slice the peppers and place in a food processor with all the other ingredients. Blend until smooth, adding water if it is too thick.

4. Serve with a sprinkle of walnuts and coriander/cilantro and a drizzle of oil. This is delicious with cucumber or carrot sticks, or spread over crackers.

HOMEMADE HARISSA

This harissa is a staple in my fridge. It's the perfect marinade for meat and is delicious in wraps. Once made you can keep it in a sealed jar for 2 weeks in the fridge.

makes 1 jar

10 fresh chillies
1½ tsp coriander seeds
½ tsp cumin seeds
½ tsp caraway seeds
4 fat garlic cloves, peeled and chopped
½ tsp sea salt
2 tsp tomato purée/paste
2½ tsp lemon juice
1 tbsp olive oil

1. Blacken the chillies on a gas hob/stovetop or lightly grill in the oven for 10 minutes. Remove from the heat and split lengthways, discarding the stalks and scraping out the seeds.

2. Toast the coriander, cumin and caraway seeds in a dry pan on a low heat until fragrant, ensuring they don't burn. Transfer the toasted seeds, together with all other ingredients into a high-speed blender and blend until a thick paste forms.

WHOLE ROASTED CAULIFLOWER

Cauliflower is the new cult dinner-party dish. I'm definitely not complaining about that; it's such a wonderful vegetable and, when it's roasted, you can see why it's finding its way onto pretty much every trendy restaurant menu. This recipe is so easy to make and is a great addition to the Middle Eastern Bowl (see pages 128–129) It also tastes delicious cold the next day, or chopped up and added to the Bodyism Frittata (see page 136). In case you hadn't guessed yet, I love cauliflower.

serves 4

1 head of cauliflower (keep the stems and
    leaves on)
120 ml/4 fl oz/½ cup olive oil
Himalayan pink salt or kosher salt (to taste)
3 tbsp toasted sesame seeds
1 tbsp chopped fresh parsley
1 tbsp chopped fresh mint
45 g/1½ oz/¼ cup pomegranate seeds

for the tahini dressing

115 g/4 oz/½ cup tahini
Juice of half a lemon
small handful of fresh coriander/cilantro
60 ml/2 fl oz/¼ cup water
half a garlic clove, peeled
salt and ground black pepper, to season

1. Preheat the oven to 180°C/350°F/gas mark 4.

2. Fill a large saucepan with water and bring to the boil. Place the cauliflower in the saucepan and leave to cook for 3 minutes.

3. Remove from the water and leave to steam dry for 10 minutes.

4. Place the cauliflower on a baking tray, drizzle all over with olive oil and season well with the salt. Roast in the preheated oven for 30–40 minutes (let it get really roasted and burnt in some places).

5. While the cauliflower is roasting, make the tahini dressing. Just place all the ingredients in a blender and whizz it up.

6. Remove the cauliflower from the oven and place on a serving plate.

7. Drizzle with the dressing and sprinkle with sesame seeds, parsley, mint and the pomegranate seeds.

HEARTY ROASTED CARROTS AND AVOCADO

This dish is inspired by one from my favourite restaurant in New York, ABC Kitchen. It looks really fresh and bright. Enjoy it with grilled fish or meat and some brown rice. Try to use multi-coloured carrots, if you can find them, but regular long carrots look lovely, too. I would advise covering your roasting trays in tin foil before putting the carrots on, to save on sticky scrubbing later (you'll thank me).

serves 4

1 tsp cumin seeds, toasted and ground (or just ground, if that's all you have)
1 tsp coriander seeds, toasted and ground (or just ground, if that's all you have)
¼ tsp sumac
1 tsp salt
2 tsp fresh thyme
4 garlic cloves, minced
¼ tsp chilli flakes
¼ tsp ground black pepper
1 tbsp red wine vinegar
4 tbsp olive oil
15 whole assorted carrots, scrubbed (there's no need to peel them)
60 ml/2 fl oz/¼ cup water
1 large avocado, cut into thin slices
2 tbsp toasted pumpkin seeds or sesame seeds
handful of any kind of sprout or rocket/arugula leaves
4 tbsp Greek yoghurt (or more, to taste)

for the dressing

1 tbsp olive oil
1 tbsp freshly squeezed lemon juice
1 tbsp freshly squeezed orange juice
pinch of salt and ground black pepper

1. Preheat the oven to 200°C/400°F/gas mark 6.

2. Make up your spice paste by grinding the cumin seeds, coriander seeds, sumac, salt and thyme in a pestle and mortar or using a small food processor. If using pre-ground spices, skip this step.

3. Put the spices in a bowl and add in the garlic, chilli, pepper, vinegar and olive oil; whisk together.

4. Spread the carrots out in a roasting pan (use two, if the carrots are too cramped). Cover them with the whisked spice mix and use your hands to make sure it's spread all over the carrots.

5. Add the water to the pan, just pouring it in around the sides of the carrots; this will help them cook. Cover the pan with tin foil wrapped tightly around it and put it into the preheated oven for 25 minutes.

6. Take the roasting pan out of the oven. The water will have evaporated. Remove the foil and put the pan back in the oven to roast for about 30 minutes. The carrots should be brown and tender, but not falling apart.

7. Meanwhile, make the dressing. Combine the olive oil, lemon juice and orange juice with the salt and pepper.

8. When the carrots are done, pour the dressing over them, then scatter the avocado, the seeds and your sprouts or rocket/arugula on top. Finish with a few dollops of yoghurt and tuck in.

SUMAC FATTOUSH

This is the Lebanese version of a chopped salad. You want to scoop the seeds out of the tomato and cucumber, or else the salad will be too wet. Make the dressing first, because the flavours will develop as it sits. This salad is wonderful paired with frankly anything, from fish and meat to vegetables. It holds up well in the fridge for a day or two.

serves 4

for the dressing

2 tsp sumac
1 tbsp warm water
1 small garlic clove, crushed
juice of half a lemon
1 tbsp extra virgin olive oil
½ tbsp white wine vinegar
pinch of salt and ground black pepper

for the salad

1 large ripe tomato, seeds removed, finely
   chopped
half a cucumber, peeled and seeds removed,
   finely chopped
1 spring onion/scallion, white and green parts,
   finely chopped
big handful of fresh parsley, leaves and stalks,
   finely chopped
handful of fresh mint, finely chopped
2 handfuls baby gem lettuce, roughly chopped

1. Make the dressing first by mixing the sumac into the warm water and leaving it to sit while you prepare the rest of the components.

2. Add the rest of the dressing ingredients, including the sumac and water, into a jam jar or bowl. Shake or whisk to mix.

3. To prepare the salad, simply add the ingredients to a bowl and mix together.

4. Pour on the dressing about 5 minutes before serving, so the vegetables retain their freshness and the dressing soaks in. Dig in!

SWEET POTATO WEDGES AND CRISPY CHICKPEA BAKE

This vegetable dish is filling enough to be a meal on its own, or you can pair it with protein, like steak or fish. The crispy baked chickpeas also make a great snack, too. Sweet potatoes are brimming with vitamins A and C and are pure comfort food.

serves 4

4 sweet potatoes
2 tbsp olive oil
1 tbsp honey
½ tsp salt
½ tsp ground black pepper
½ tsp crushed red pepper flakes
1 x 400-g/14-oz can chickpeas, drained, rinsed and dried with a clean tea towel (the drier the chickpeas are before baking, the more they'll crisp up in the oven!)
¼ tsp smoked paprika
¼ tsp ground cumin
handful of fresh coriander/cilantro, chopped

for the yoghurt dressing

¼ tub organic Greek yoghurt
1 spring onion/scallion, chopped
2 tbsp freshly squeezed lime juice (or more, to taste)
salt and ground black pepper (optional)

1. Preheat your oven to 200°C/400°F/gas mark 6.

2. Cover 2 baking trays with tin foil — one for the chickpeas and one for the sweet potatoes.

3. Wash and pat dry the sweet potatoes — you don't need to peel them. Chop lengthways into large, long wedges. Lay them on one of the foil-covered trays and drizzle with a tablespoon of olive oil and the honey, then sprinkle over ¼ teaspoon each of salt and pepper and the red pepper flakes. Toss to coat, then arrange them in an even layer.

4. Put the baking tray on the top shelf of the oven and cook for 40 minutes, or until cooked through.

5. Pour the chickpeas into the other foil-covered tray and drizzle over a tablespoon of the olive oil, then sprinkle with the smoked paprika, cumin and the remaining salt and pepper.

6. Mix everything together, spreading the chickpeas into an even layer, and put on the bottom shelf of the oven for about 30 minutes. After 12 minutes, give them a toss to ensure even cooking.

7. Meanwhile, make the yoghurt dressing. Whisk the yoghurt, spring onion/scallion and lime juice together. Add a sprinkle of salt and pepper, if desired.

8. Pour the chickpeas over the sweet potatoes. Add dollops of the yoghurt on top and sprinkle with chopped coriander/cilantro for a fresh kick.

DESSERTS

CHERRY COBBLER

The cherries give this dessert such a lovely sweetness, which, mixed with the sponge, is pretty special. This is obviously an indulgent dessert, so please don't think you are being 'kind to yourself' if you have it every day — but, when you do have it, enjoy it!

serves 8–10

115 g/4 oz/½ cup butter

75 g/2⅔ oz/generous ½ cup brown rice flour

50 g/1¾ oz/½ cup buckwheat flour

50 g/1¾ oz/½ cup ground almonds, plus an extra 1 tbsp for the cherries

100 g/3½ oz/½ cup coconut palm sugar, plus 1 tbsp for the top

zest of 1 lemon

1 tsp baking powder

235 ml/8 fl oz/1 cup almond milk

310 g/11 oz/1½ cups pitted cherries, fresh or frozen

1. Preheat the oven to 180°C/350°F/gas mark 4.

2. Grease a 20 x 30-cm/8 x 12-inch baking dish. Melt the butter in a small saucepan.

3. Mix the flours, ground almonds, coconut palm sugar, lemon zest and baking powder in a big mixing bowl. Stir in the melted butter and almond milk until thoroughly mixed.

4. Pour the mixture into the baking dish.

5. Place the cherries in a bowl and toss with the extra tablespoon of ground almonds. Scatter the cherry mixture evenly over the mix in the dish. Do not stir it!

6. Sprinkle with the remaining tablespoon of coconut palm sugar and bake for 40 minutes in the preheated oven, until it goes lovely and golden brown. A skewer should come out clean when poked into the centre.

MY APPLE AND MULBERRY CRUMBLE

When the apples are falling off the trees at the end of the summer, I make this with the kids. Sunday afternoons go up a gear when a crumble is cooking in the oven. As always, you are in charge, so if apples aren't your thing then swap them for pears, or lose a few apples and replace them with berries. Enjoy with a scoop of Bodyism ice-cream (see Bodyism Sundae on page 205).

serves 6

6 apples, cored and chopped (choose any variety; I like Braeburn best)
juice of 1 lemon
1 tbsp coconut palm sugar or honey
1 tsp vanilla extract
100 g/3½ oz/⅔ cup dried mulberries

for the topping

40 g/1½ oz/¼ cup hazelnuts, toasted
90 g/3 oz/1 cup gluten-free oats
50 g/1¾ oz/½ cup ground almonds
40 g/1½ oz/½ cup flaked/slivered almonds
½ tsp Himalayan pink salt
1 tbsp xylitol
½ tsp ground cinnamon
½ tsp vanilla extract
3 tbsp coconut oil, melted
2 tbsp maple syrup

1. Preheat the oven to 180°C/350°F/gas mark 4.

2. Place the apples in a large saucepan and heat over a low heat. Add the lemon juice, coconut palm sugar or honey, vanilla extract and mulberries. Let the mixture cook until softened — approximately 15 minutes.

3. Meanwhile, make the topping. In a food processor, blitz the hazelnuts into a crumb consistency. Pour into a mixing bowl.

4. Add the oats, ground almonds, flaked/slivered almonds, salt, xylitol and cinnamon and mix well.

5. In a separate bowl, mix the vanilla extract, coconut oil and maple syrup and stir. Slowly add the wet mixture into the dry mixture and mix well.

6. Lay the crumble mix on a baking tray and use a spatula to pat it down so that it is densely packed.

7. Bake for 15 minutes in the preheated oven, until the crumble has started to golden slightly. Remove from the oven and leave to cool.

8. Pour the apple mixture into an ovenproof gratin dish. Using the spatula again, place the crumble mix on top of the apple mixture.

9. Bake for 15 minutes, but keep an eye on the oven. If the crumble browns too quickly, cover it with tin foil for the remaining cooking time.

COCONUT CARROT CAKE

This is the best free-from cake I have ever made — the coconut icing/frosting is so delicious and creamy, and goes perfectly with the lightness of the sponge. It's really important you use a good-quality, full-fat coconut milk. If you use one that is branded 'light', then it's likely the added ingredients will mean it won't separate, which is essential for this recipe.

The coconut milk needs to be put in the fridge the night before and the bowl you whisk it in needs to be chilled beforehand, but, apart from that, this cake is really simple and easy to make for any occasion.

serves 10

for the sponge

3 tbsp coconut milk (use just the cream from the top of the can in the fridge)
150 g/5¼ oz/¾ cup virgin coconut oil, melted
3 organic, free-range eggs, yolks and whites separated
1 tsp vanilla extract
100 g/3½ oz/½ cup coconut palm sugar
70 g/2½ oz/¾ cup desiccated/dried shredded coconut
180 g/6⅓ oz/3½ cups carrots, grated
½ tsp salt
2 tsp ground cinnamon
1 tsp baking powder
½ tsp bicarbonate of soda/baking soda
150 g/5¼ oz/1¼ cups self-raising/self-rising gluten-free flour

for the icing/frosting and topping

1 x 400-ml/14-fl oz can full-fat coconut milk
1 tbsp rice malt syrup
½ tsp vanilla extract
1 tsp ground cinnamon, plus extra for sprinkling
handful of chopped walnuts

1. Put the coconut milk in the fridge the night before you make the cake, and put a mixing bowl in the fridge to chill, too.

2. Next, grease the sides of a 20-cm/8-inch circular cake tin and line the base with parchment paper. Preheat the oven to 180°C/350°F/gas mark 4.

3. Put 3 tablespoons of coconut milk, the melted coconut oil, egg yolks and vanilla extract into a mixing bowl (not the one in the fridge), and whisk together until combined.

4. Mix together the coconut palm sugar, desiccated/dried shredded coconut, carrots, salt, cinnamon, baking powder and bicarbonate of soda/baking soda and flour until well combined. Add the coconut milk mixture and whisk together until no lumps remain.

5. Whisk the egg whites in a separate bowl until they are stiff and remain in the bowl when it is held upside down.

6. Fold the egg whites into the cake mixture with a metal spoon. 'Fold' is the key word, here. You want to get as much air into the cake as possible to make it light and fluffy.

7. Pour the mixture into the cake tin and place in the preheated oven. Bake for 35–40 minutes, or until an inserted skewer comes out clean.

8. While the cake is in the oven, start making the coconut icing/frosting. Place the thick cream from the can of coconut milk into the chilled mixing bowl. Add in the rice malt syrup and vanilla extract and whisk until the cream looks smooth and fluffy. Set aside in the fridge to firm up.

9. When the cake has finished in the oven, leave it to cool in the tin for 5 minutes, then turn it out onto a wire rack and leave to cool. Once fully cool, spread an even layer of icing/frosting on the cake.

10. Dust with extra cinnamon and sprinkle the chopped walnuts on the top.

PERSIAN LOVE CAKE

This delicious spiced dessert is the perfect celebration cake, dinner-party dessert or scrumptious treat. The Middle Eastern spices give it a rich, complex flavour, which, combined with the gooey texture, creates an indulgent, satisfying cake. Serve this with a spoon of Greek yoghurt (ideally to someone you love, or fancy) as a whole lot of love goes into this cake.

serves 6-8

180 g/6⅓ oz/2 cups ground almonds
250 g/8¾ oz/1¼ cups coconut palm sugar
½ tsp Himalayan pink salt
80 g/2¾ oz/⅓ cup unsalted butter, chilled
1 organic, free-range egg
125 g/4½ oz/½ cup organic Greek yoghurt, plus extra to serve
½ tsp ground cinnamon
½ tsp ground nutmeg
½ tsp ground cardamom
2 tbsp shelled pistachios, roughly chopped
2 tbsp edible rose petals, to garnish (not essential, but beautiful)

1. Preheat the oven to 180°C/350°F/gas mark 4.

2. Grease the sides of an 18-cm/7-inch spring-form cake tin and line the base with parchment paper.

3. Mix the almond meal, sugar and salt in a bowl to combine evenly. Add the chilled butter and rub with your fingertips until the mixture resembles coarse breadcrumbs.

4. Spoon half the mixture into the prepared tin and press down firmly to cover the base evenly, as if you were making a cheesecake.

5. Add the egg, yoghurt and spices to the remaining mixture and beat with a wooden spoon until smooth and creamy. Pour this mixture over the prepared base and sprinkle the chopped pistachios around the edge of the cake.

6. Bake until golden brown and just set, approximately 30 minutes.

7. Allow to cool completely in the tin on a wire rack, before removing from the tin and transferring to a serving plate.

8. Sprinkle with rose petals (if using) and serve with an extra dollop of Greek yoghurt on the side.

HONEY CAKE

This is one of Chrissy's favourites. The texture of the cake is so moist and we love it with a big pot of coffee. If blueberries aren't your thing, swap them for another berry or any fruit of your choice.

serves 8–10

4 tbsp good-quality olive oil, plus extra for greasing
240 g/8½ oz/2 cups ground almonds
1 tsp baking powder
½ tsp bicarbonate of soda/baking soda
½ tsp ground cinnamon
½ tsp ground ginger
½ tsp Himalayan pink salt
3 organic, free-range eggs, beaten
235 g/8⅓ oz/⅔ cup acacia honey, plus an extra 1 tbsp for the glaze
1 lemon (zest and juice)
170 g/6 oz/1¾ cups blueberries
50 g/1¾ oz/½ cup toasted pistachios, chopped

1. Preheat the oven to 180°C/350°F/gas mark 4. Using olive oil, grease the sides of a 23-cm/9-inch spring-form cake tin and line the base with parchment paper.

2. Mix together the ground almonds, baking powder, bicarbonate of soda/baking soda, cinnamon, ginger and salt.

3. Mix together the beaten eggs, honey, olive oil and lemon zest. Add to the dry ingredients and mix well, until combined, then gently fold in the blueberries. Pour the mixture into the prepared cake tin.

4. Bake for 55 minutes–1 hour in the preheated oven, until the cake is deeply golden brown and the centre is firm to the touch (and a skewer inserted into the middle comes out clean). If the top of the cake browns too quickly, just cover it with tin foil and bake for the remaining time. Leave the cake in its tin and place on a wire rack to cool.

5. Slice the lemon in half and squeeze out the juice from both halves. Combine the lemon juice with the extra honey in a small saucepan and warm over a low heat. Stir until well combined. Brush the glaze over the warm cake.

6. Once the cake is cool, remove it from the tin and sprinkle with the chopped pistachios and serve.

MOLTEN CHOCOLATE POTS

I love a chocolate pudding. This molten pot is extremely indulgent and has all the satisfaction, without all the sugar. The outside edge holds it shape and, when you cut into the middle, the chocolate oozes out. For this recipe, you will need two large ramekins or three smaller ones.

serves 2–3

50 g/1¾ oz/½ cup cacao powder, plus extra to dust
2 tbsp arrowroot powder
1 tbsp xylitol
1 tsp vanilla bean powder
100 g/3½ oz coconut oil, plus extra for greasing
2 tbsp cacao butter
155 g/5½ oz/⅔ cup maple syrup
2 organic, free-range eggs, plus 1 additional yolk
¼ tsp Himalayan pink salt

1. Preheat the oven to 180°C/350°F/gas mark 4.

2. In a bowl, combine the cacao, arrowroot, xylitol and vanilla powder, and set aside.

3. Put a small saucepan over a low heat and melt the coconut oil, cacao butter and maple syrup. Once melted and combined, pour into the dry ingredients and mix well.

4. Add the two whole eggs and additional yolk and whisk to incorporate.

5. Grease and line the ramekins with coconut oil and spoon in the mixture. Place in the fridge for 10–15 minutes.

6. Once chilled, bake for 10 minutes in the preheated oven. Remove and let stand for 1 minute.

7. Ease them out of the ramekins onto plates and dust with cacao powder.

BODYISM SUNDAE

I've always had a thing for ice-cream. As I've got older and more in tune with my body, I've realized that a mountain of ice-cream makes me hysterical — I can't handle all that sugar. So, when I discovered how easy it is to make ice-cream that is just as delicious, without all the unnecessary, toxic, refined sugar, I felt (and continue to feel) extremely smug. Now I'm sharing my secret. The trick here is to remember it's all about the toppings, so pile it high (and mindfully) with all the extras.

serves 4

4 bananas, peeled, sliced and frozen
2 tbsp rice milk
1 scoop Bodyism Protein Excellence (or, if you want a stronger chocolate flavour, go for Body Brilliance) — if you don't have the supplements, then don't worry!
1 tbsp cacao
1 tsp ground cinnamon
2 tbsp almond butter
pinch of salt

for the toppings
Simply Granola (see page 102)
cacao nibs
toasted coconut flakes
goji berries
mulberries
chunks of Bodyism Cookies, if you want extra indulgence (see page 176)
The list could go on and on!

1. In a blender, mix the bananas and rice milk until you have a smooth consistency.

2. Add the Bodyism supplement, cacao, cinnamon, almond butter and salt. Mix again.

3. Transfer to a freezer-proof container and freeze for 1 hour.

4. Scoop and serve, covered with all the toppings!

GRILLED FIGS WITH GREEK YOGHURT AND MANUKA HONEY

This is such a simple dessert, but whenever I make it, it reminds me that, if you choose delicious, good-quality ingredients, you don't need to do anything fancy with them. This is a light, refreshing yet wholesome treat. If you like fruit for breakfast, then you can definitely include this as a breakfast option (although I'd add some Bodyism Protein Excellence to the yoghurt, just so you get a good dose of protein to give you energy for the day).

serves 4

4 large figs
2 tsp ground cinnamon
1 tsp maple syrup (optional)
handful of rosemary sprigs
8 tbsp coconut yoghurt
2 tbsp pecans, chopped and toasted

1. Preheat the oven to 180°C/350°F/gas mark 4 and line a baking tray with parchment paper.

2. Slice the figs into halves and quarters. Place them on the prepared baking tray.

3. Sprinkle 1 teaspoon of the cinnamon over the figs and drizzle with the maple syrup. Lastly, lay the rosemary sprigs over the figs, too.

4. Place in the preheated oven for approximately 40 minutes, until caramelized and soft. Leave to cool for 10 minutes.

5. Serve each fig with 2 tablespoons of the coconut yoghurt and sprinkle with the pecans and the remaining teaspoon of cinnamon.

BERRY COCONUT ICE LOLLIES

These are the kids' absolute favourite. Use this recipe as a guide and swap the fruit and milk as you wish! You will need standard ice-lolly moulds for this recipe.

makes 12

150 g/5¼ oz/1½ cups blueberries, frozen
   or fresh
1½ tbsp water
3 tbsp maple syrup
1 scoop Bodyism Berry Burn
175 ml/6¼ fl oz/¾ cup canned coconut milk
120 ml/4 fl oz/½ cup almond milk

1. In a small saucepan, combine the blueberries, water and maple syrup. Bring to the boil and cook over a low heat until it becomes quite thick. Remove from the heat.

2. In a small bowl, whisk together the Berry Burn, coconut milk and almond milk.

3. Pour the milk mixture into the ice-lolly moulds until they are half full. Spoon in the blueberry mixture to fill each mould.

4. Place in the freezer for 1 hour and then insert the wooden sticks into each ice-lolly.

5. Place the moulds back in the freezer for another 5 hours (until they have become solid lollies).

SPELT CRUST PLUM PIE

Victoria plums are beautifully sweet when they are in season and there is nothing better than a delicious summer fruit pie served with a dollop of ice cream (see Bodyism Sundae on page 205).

serves 8
for the pastry
200 g/7 oz/⅔ cup cold, organic butter, cubed, plus extra for greasing
300 g/10½ oz/2⅓ cups light spelt flour or plain flour/all-purpose flour, plus extra for dusting
2 tbsp coconut palm sugar
pinch of salt
2 organic, free-range eggs

for the filling
900 g/2 lb/5 cups ripe plums
4 tbsp maple syrup
2 tbsp cornflour/cornstarch
1 tsp ground cinnamon

1. Grease a 20-cm/8-inch pie dish with butter and dust with flour. Preheat the oven to 180°C/350°F/gas mark 4.

2. To make the pastry, mix together the flour, half the coconut sugar and salt in a bowl. Rub in the butter using your fingertips until it resembles fine breadcrumbs, then stir in one of the eggs and press the mixture together to make a ball of dough. Wrap the dough in clingfilm/plastic wrap and put it in the fridge for 30 minutes.

3. For the filling, cut the plums in half and take out the stones. Mix with the maple syrup, cornflour/cornstarch and cinnamon. Let sit for a couple of minutes so that the cornflour can dissolve.

4. Remove the dough from the fridge and divide it into two pieces. Roll out one half on a floured surface until large enough to line the pie dish. Place the pastry in the dish, pressing it into the base and up the sides then trim the top to give a neat edge. Line the pastry with parchment paper, fill with baking beans and blind bake in the oven for 10–15 minutes until starting to turn golden. Remove the parchment and beans from the case and add the plum filling.

5. Whisk the remaining egg and brush it lightly over the sides of the pastry case.

6. Roll out the remaining pastry and cut it into thin strips. Make a criss-cross pattern on top of the pie with the pastry strips, pressing the ends to the sides to seal. Brush the pastry top with egg, then sprinkle with the remaining coconut sugar.

7. Bake the pie in the preheated oven for about 45 minutes, until the pastry is golden and the filling is bubbling. Remove from the oven and leave it to cool completely before serving.

COMFORTING COCONUT RICE PUDDING

This is an old-school classic I grew up loving. My mum was way ahead of her time in her knowledge of healthy eating; she always tried to use whole, unprocessed ingredients, even when we didn't have a lot of money to spend. You can certainly make it with dairy alternatives, but if you fancy something lighter and dairy free, make it as instructed below. I love rice pudding with a dollop of fruit compote or some berries and flaked/slivered almonds — it's all down to personal preference.

serves 6

500 ml/17 fl oz/2 cups water
500 ml/17 fl oz/2 cups rice milk
1 x 400-ml/14-fl oz can coconut milk
2 tbsp honey
1 whole vanilla pod/bean
6 cardamom pods
3 tbsp desiccated/dried shredded coconut
300 g/10½ oz/1⅔ cups short-grain brown rice
½ tbsp lemon zest
pinch of salt

1. Pour the water, rice milk, coconut milk and honey into a heavy-bottomed pot. Turn the heat on to medium and allow the mix to slowly come up to a simmer.

2. In the meantime, split the vanilla pod/bean lengthways and scrape the seeds out with a sharp knife. Add the seeds and pod/bean into the liquid.

3. Crush the cardamom pods in a pestle and mortar or with the back of a knife, and add them to the liquid as well. Bear in mind that you can fish out the pods later, if desired.

4. Add in the desiccated/dried shredded coconut, the rice, lemon zest and the salt. Turn the heat down and allow this mixture to gently simmer for about 1 hour, stirring regularly so the rice doesn't clump together or burn.

5. Preheat the oven to 190°C/375°F/gas mark 5. Once the liquid has reduced and the rice is basically cooked, pour the mixture into a shallow dish and put it in the oven for 15 minutes to firm up.

6. Take it out and cover the top of the dish with clingfilm/plastic wrap, ensuring the plastic touches the top of the pudding so that a skin cannot form.

7. Refrigerate until completely cool and set. Serve with compote, berries, ice-cream or whatever you like!

SUPER SEAWEED PANNA COTTA

Irish seaweed, or carrageen moss, is world-renowned for its health properties and is a traditional remedy I grew up with for colds and flu. Normally made with dairy milk, this recipe is a vegan version. It takes minutes to make and keeps in the fridge for a few days, so it is the perfect make-ahead or last-minute healthy dessert. Serve with berries or fruit compote and a drizzle of honey.

serves 4
handful of dried carrageen moss
1 x 400-ml/14-fl oz can coconut milk
1 vanilla pod/bean, split lengthways and
   seeds scraped out
1 tbsp honey

1. Run the handful of dried seaweed under cold water for a minute to rehydrate.

2. Put it into a pot with the coconut milk, vanilla seeds and the split vanilla pod/bean and gently heat to a low simmer. Don't boil it. Keep an eye on it and watch the liquid thicken for about 7 minutes, stirring it every so often with a wooden spoon.

3. Pour the liquid through a fine-mesh sieve/strainer into whatever bowl or little ramekins you plan to serve the Super Seaweed Panna Cotta in. Add the honey and stir.

4. Let the liquid cool and put it into the fridge to set for 1–2 hours.

5. Once set, it is firm and has a panna-cotta-like consistency (it will wobble slightly when shaken).

6. Serve with whatever toppings you like; it's lovely with fruit compote and crunchy seeds.

THE ONLY RUB YOU'LL EVER NEED

We all need a failsafe rub recipe for those nights when we're cooking something basic, but are craving flavour. Make double or triple the quantity and store it in a jar, ready to whip out at the last minute.

serves 4

2 tbsp whole cumin seeds
2 tbsp whole coriander seeds
1 tbsp ground cinnamon
2 tsp ground ginger
1 tsp freshly ground black pepper
1 tsp ground turmeric

1. Toast all of the spices, both whole and ground together, in a dry pan for 2–3 minutes, until fragrant. If you only have pre-ground spices, then still follow this step.

2. Put everything together in a spice grinder or pestle and mortar and grind to a powder, unless you only had pre-ground spices to begin with.

3. Put the ground mix into a jar, where it will keep for up to 6 months, or add a pinch of salt and cover whatever chicken or meat you're cooking, for aromatic flavour.

THE ONLY MARINADE YOU'LL EVER NEED

A delicious marinade is the way to give your meat, fish or tempeh the x-factor. Learn this recipe so that you're safe if you're pushed for time but don't want to compromise on flavour.

serves 4

1 tbsp Dijon mustard
juice of half a lemon
½ tsp smoked paprika
¼ tsp salt
¼ tsp ground black pepper
3 tbsp olive oil

1. Mix the mustard, lemon juice, smoked paprika, salt and pepper in a bowl. Slowly whisk in the olive oil so it emulsifies nicely into a creamy mix.

2. Pour this mix over chicken or potatoes before cooking, for a smoky, uplifting taste.

THE ONLY SALAD DRESSING YOU'LL EVER NEED

This basic salad dressing is my weeknight staple, perfect over any type of salad. For a twist, simply swap out the white wine vinegar for balsamic. Make a big batch and it will keep in the fridge for up to 5 days.

serves 4

2 tbsp extra virgin olive oil
2 tbsp water
1 tbsp apple cider vinegar
1 tsp lemon juice
1 tsp tahini
1 tsp tamari
½ Dijon mustard
pinch of salt and ground black pepper

1. Put all the ingredients into a bowl or clean jam jar and shake or whisk until the dressing forms a smooth, emulsified consistency.

2. Taste it and make the dressing your own by adding more lemon juice, a shallot or a dash more vinegar.

3. Pour over salad leaves, toss together and serve.

Top Tip Add in some finely chopped shallot or garlic for a more pronounced flavour.

BEAUTY FOOD

Our Beauty Food skin-and-hair supplement is an all-natural daily elixir of super greens and marine collagen peptides, which can help prevent ageing skin and will give you that much-needed glow. This is my take on the less impressive 'green juice'.

serves 1

1 scoop Bodyism Beauty Food
5-cm/2-inch piece of cucumber, peeled
juice of half a lime
355 ml/12 fl oz/1½ cups coconut water
2 sprigs of fresh mint
100 g/3½ oz ice

1. Just whizz it up in a blender and enjoy!

ULTIMATE CLEAN

This shake is a high-fibre probiotic formula, which contains slippery elm, wild rosella and rice bran, and is flavoured with raw cacao, carob and vanilla. The formula supports gut health by cleansing your insides and helps to keep you regular!

serves 1

1 scoop Bodyism Ultimate Clean
half an avocado
355 ml/12 fl oz/1½ cups brown rice milk
1 sprig of fresh mint
100 g/3½ oz ice

1. Just whizz it up in a blender and enjoy!

BODY BRILLIANCE

Our Body Brilliance supplement is an all-natural vegan protein supplement, which is packed with super greens, minerals, energizing herbs, fruit and vegetables. We call it the 'supermodel's secret weapon'.

serves 1
1 scoop Bodyism Body Brilliance
1 tbsp almond butter
355 ml/12 fl oz/1½ cups almond milk
1 tbsp cacao
1 shot of espresso or 2 tbsp brewed coffee
100 g/3½ oz ice

1. Just whizz it up in a blender and enjoy!

BERRY BURN

This is a deliciously thick post-workout shake, perfect for muscle recovery. Berry Burn is made with a range of different berries which are packed with antioxidants.

serves 1

100 ml/3½ fl oz coconut milk
200 ml/7 fl oz coconut water
1 scoop Bodyism Berry Burn
100 g/3½ oz/1 cup frozen blueberries
1 heaped tbsp chia seeds
1 tbsp smooth almond butter

1. Just whizz it up in a blender and enjoy!

CHAI CASHEW MYLK

This is better than my childhood memories of warm milk and honey. The mix of spices reminds me of a cold winter's evening, which is why I love to make this for the kids and me to enjoy in front of a movie, with some Bodyism ice-cream (see Bodyism Sundae on page 205). If you have the Bodyism Serenity supplement, try adding one scoop to the recipe.

serves 4

for the cashew mylk

125 g/4½ oz/1 cup cashews
950 ml/1⅔ pints/4 cups filtered water
a couple of pinches of Himalayan pink salt
1 tsp raw honey
3 tsp ground cinnamon
2 tsp vanilla powder or extract

for the chai spice mix

½ tsp ground black pepper
2 tbsp ground cinnamon
2 tbsp ground ginger
1 tbsp ground cardamom
1 tbsp ground cloves
½ tbsp ground nutmeg

1. Soak the cashews overnight in a large sealed jar with half the water and a pinch of Himalayan pink salt.

2. In the morning, drain the liquid and wash the cashews in a sieve/strainer, until the water runs clear. Add to a blender with all the other Cashew Mylk ingredients and the remaining water. Blend for 3 minutes. Check the creaminess and add more water, if it's too thick.

3. Now make the Chai Spice Mix. Combine all the spices together in a pestle and mortar and sift through a fine-mesh sieve/strainer. If you are using whole spices, make sure the ground mixture is very fine. Put in a sealed jar and enjoy for up to 1 week after making it. The Chai Spice Mix can also be used to make a delicious warming tea.

4. To make the Chai Cashew Mylk, add 1 tablespoon of Chai Spice Mix to the blender and blend again. Pour through a sieve/strainer into a bottle and keep for up to 4 days in the fridge.

INDEX

Publisher's acknowledgements

Cover photography by Julie
Adams and Kate Davis-Mcleod.
Photography on pages 2–93 by
Kate Davis-Mcleod and on pages
94–221 by David Munns.
Copy editing by Daniella Isaacs.
Recipe development by Julia
Harvey, Daniella Isaacs and
Rachael McKeon.

FINAL WORDS

Here's the bad news...

Reading a book on how to change your life will not make a difference. Only you can make the difference. You can't plead ignorance anymore because the power is in your hands. You need to be kind to yourself.

Here's the good news...

From this very moment on, you have everything you need to completely transform your life, your health, your body, your thoughts... everything.

Remember, your past does not equal your future. Look at every past diet you've tried as a lesson which has made you stronger and more powerful. There is no such thing as failure — only feedback.

Knowing isn't enough — it's doing. You have an in-built, infallible guide within you, that loves you, that cares for you and that knows you better than anyone else — that is you. You are your best expert.

Our bodies are incredible, magical and wonderful. The problem is, we've been taught to mistrust ourselves, to numb ourselves through medication, toxic food, screen addiction and any number of other distractions. This numbness brings us no joy, no happiness and no comfort. We are uncomfortably numb. This book will introduce you to the most sophisticated, powerful, highly tuned technology ever created: you. Start with the two-week programme, then learn to trust yourself.

Final three thoughts...

1. Let go of shame and guilt.
2. Trust yourself.
3. Be unstoppable.

And one more thing: make your world impeccable. If you say you're going to do something, do it.

Thank yous...

As always there are so many beautiful people to thank. None of this would be possible without the incredible, selfless contribution of so many wonderful people.

To Chrissy and Nat, you're a constant source of strength and inspiration.

To my friend. partner, mentor and big brother, Ferit, thank you for believing in me and thank you for making everything and anything possible. Thank you Tevfik for your unwavering support in everything we do. To Tom Koenig, for eating all the cheese toasties, and Luke and Chantelle, for always being there no matter what. Thank you Adrian at Kruger Crowne, for making this all happen.

To our wonderful contributors; Rhaya, thank you for your intelligence, kindness and genius — your passion and commitment is incredible. To Matt Bevan, for helping with the exercises and for being supremely dedicated. To Daniella, Rachael and Julia, for the delicious recipes.

To everyone from the greatest team in the history of the universe, Bodyism, thank you for your dedication, positivity and drive. To all of the people that have supported us over the past 10 years; our clients, our customers, our members, thank you so much.

To Emily Ezekiel, David Munns, Kitty Coles and India Whiley-Morton, for making our delicious food look even more amazing. To Kate Davis-Macleod, our shoot at the D-Hotel was incredible and made us feel extremely lucky. Thanks also to Julie Adams.

And, thanks for my dad, for watching over me and making everything seem okay.

This is for my children.